W9-CGZ-489

WITHDRAWN

Also Available From the American Academy of Pediatrics

Common Conditions

Allergies and Asthma: What Every Parent Needs to Know

The Big Book of Symptoms: A–Z Guide to Your
   Child's Health

Mama Doc Medicine: Finding Calm and Confidence
   in Parenting, Child Health, and Work-Life Balance

My Child Is Sick! Expert Advice for Managing
   Common Illnesses and Injuries

Sleep: What Every Parent Needs to Know

Waking Up Dry: A Guide to Help Children
   Overcome Bedwetting

Developmental, Behavioral, and Psychosocial Information

ADHD: What Every Parent Needs to Know

Autism Spectrum Disorders: What Every Parent
   Needs to Know

CyberSafe: Protecting and Empowering Kids in
   the Digital World of Texting, Gaming, and
   Social Media

Mental Health, Naturally: The Family Guide to
   Holistic Care for a Healthy Mind and Body

Newborns, Infants, and Toddlers

Baby Care Anywhere: A Quick Guide to Parenting
   On the Go

Caring for Your Baby and Young Child: Birth to Age 5*

Dad to Dad: Parenting Like a Pro

Guide to Toilet Training*

Heading Home With Your Newborn:
   From Birth to Reality

Mommy Calls: Dr. Tanya Answers Parents' Top
   101 Questions About Babies and Toddlers

New Mother's Guide to Breastfeeding*

Raising Twins: Parenting Multiples From Pregnancy
   Through the School Years

Retro Baby: Cut Back on All the Gear and Boost
   Your Baby's Development With More Than
   100 Time-tested Activities

Your Baby's First Year*

Nutrition and Fitness

Food Fights: Winning the Nutritional Challenges
   of Parenthood Armed With Insight, Humor,
   and a Bottle of Ketchup

Nutrition: What Every Parent Needs to Know

A Parent's Guide to Childhood Obesity:
   A Road Map to Health

The Picky Eater Project: 6 Weeks to Happier,
   Healthier Family Mealtimes

Sports Success R_x! Your Child's Prescription for
   the Best Experience

School-aged Children and Adolescents

Building Resilience in Children and Teens:
   Giving Kids Roots and Wings

Raising Kids to Thrive: Balancing Love With
   Expectations and Protection With Trust

For additional parenting resources, visit the HealthyChildren bookstore at

shop.aap.org/for-parents.

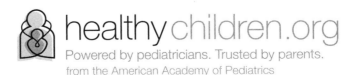

healthychildren.org
Powered by pediatricians. Trusted by parents.
from the American Academy of Pediatrics

*This book is also available in Spanish.

Understanding the NICU

What Parents of Preemies and Other Hospitalized Newborns Need to Know

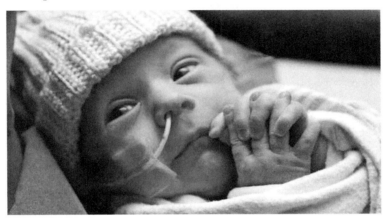

Jeanette Zaichkin, RN, MN, NNP-BC, Editor in Chief

Gary Weiner, MD, FAAP, Contributing Editor

David Loren, MD, FAAP, Contributing Editor

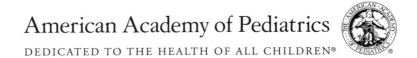

American Academy of Pediatrics

DEDICATED TO THE HEALTH OF ALL CHILDREN®

American Academy of Pediatrics Publishing Staff

Mark Grimes, *Director, Department of Publishing*
Kathryn Sparks, *Manager, Consumer Publishing*
Holly Kaminski, *Editor, Consumer Publishing*
Shannan Martin, *Production Manager, Consumer Publications*
Jason Crase, *Manager, Editorial Services*
Linda Diamond, *Manager, Art Direction and Production*
Mary Lou White, *Director, Department of Marketing and Sales*
Sara Hoerdeman, *Marketing Manager, Consumer Products*

About the American Academy of Pediatrics

The American Academy of Pediatrics is an organization of 66,000 primary care pediatricians, pediatric medical subspecialists, and pediatric surgical specialists dedicated to the health, safety, and well-being of infants, children, adolescents, and young adults.

Published by the American Academy of Pediatrics
141 Northwest Point Blvd
Elk Grove Village, IL 60007-1019
Telephone: 847/434-4000
Fax: 847/434-8000
www.aap.org

The information contained in this publication should not be used as a substitute for the medical care and advice of your pediatrician. There may be variations in treatment that your pediatrician may recommend based on individual facts and circumstances.

Statements and opinions expressed are those of the authors and not necessarily those of the American Academy of Pediatrics.

Listing of resources does not imply an endorsement by the American Academy of Pediatrics (AAP). The AAP is not responsible for the content of external resources. Information was current at the time of publication.

Brand names are furnished for identification purposes only. No endorsement of the manufacturers or products mentioned is implied.

This publication has been developed by the American Academy of Pediatrics. The contributors are expert authorities in the field of pediatrics. No commercial involvement of any kind has been solicited or accepted in development of the content of this publication. Disclosure: David Loren has equity interest (stock) in the following companies: Abbott Laboratories, Abbvie Inc, Bristol Myers Squibb Co, The Cooper Companies Inc, Johnson & Johnson, Varian Medical Systems, Medtronic, Novo-Nordisk, Stryker Corp, and Teva Pharmaceutical.

Except where noted, the photographs in this publication were provided by families as a visual representation of their personal NICU experiences and do not necessarily depict American Academy of Pediatrics policy. Every effort is made to keep *Understanding the NICU* consistent with the most recent advice and information available from the American Academy of Pediatrics.

The publishers have made every effort to trace the copyright holders for borrowed material. If they have inadvertently overlooked any, they will be pleased to make the necessary arrangements at the first opportunity.

Special discounts are available for bulk purchases of this publication. E-mail our Special Sales Department at aapsales@aap.org for more information.

Printed in the United States of America
9-373   1 2 3 4 5 6 7 8 9 10
CB0098
ISBN: 978-1-61002-048-0
eBook: 978-1-61002-049-7
Cover photography by Gigi O'Dea, memoryportraitsbygigi.com. Used by permission.
Library of Congress Control Number: 2015960373

What People Are Saying

Once again, Jeanette Zaichkin has demonstrated her gift for empathizing with and educating the parents of a premature or sick baby in the NICU.

Over the past several decades, neonatology has evolved from a relatively primitive subspecialty of pediatrics to a well-evidenced science on its own, involving highly technical equipment and medical interventions that can create seeming miracles when viewed from a distance. However, the neonatal intensive care unit can be frightening, confusing, and often an overwhelming experience for the parents of a critically ill newly born baby. In many cases, this temporary home has been thrust on parents without warning, at a time when they had been looking forward to a beautiful, intimate, and very personal event for their family. Jeanette and her colleagues have written an articulate, sensitive, empathetic, and very accurate book that will help pave the way for parents as they and their newborn find themselves living in the NICU for weeks and often even months.

Jeanette's book gives parents the tools to become better informed during this scary time. The book untangles medical terminology and hospital procedures that are often frightening for a parent. Jeanette explains the multiple roles of hospital staff involved in their baby's care. She includes family stories and direct quotes, allowing the reader to feel less alone in a time of crisis. Feelings of powerlessness and helplessness are often overwhelming emotions, making it difficult for parents to bond with and comfort their baby. The book acknowledges these frustrations, encourages parents to ask thoughtful questions, worry less, and therefore to become more involved with their baby's care.

The authors of this book are highly qualified. Jeanette is well recognized for her superb teaching expertise as she provided the nursing perspective to help guide the evolution of the Neonatal Resuscitation Program over the past 18 years. And Gary Weiner and David Loren, both well-seasoned neonatologists, have validated the authenticity of the medical content, as well as providing the neonatologist's perspective. Gary is editor of the new *Textbook of Neonatal Resuscitation*.

In summary, we can highly recommend this new book for the parents of a NICU baby, but also to the nurses, physicians, and allied staff in the NICU, to help remind them of the perspective of the parents whenever a new high-risk baby is admitted to their unit.

John Kattwinkel, MD, FAAP
Professor Emeritus, Neonatal Intensive Care Unit, University of Virginia

Sarah M. Wilson, MSN, NNP-BC
Advance Practice Nurse 2, Neonatal Intensive Care Unit, University of Virginia

—◦◦◦—

Understanding the NICU provides a much-needed resource for families thrust into the unfamiliar world of neonatal intensive care. The parent stories woven into this book help parents to relate and to have hope. The book is well written, easy to follow with lots of boxes and tables to provide quick easy-to-follow pointers for parents. A must-have resource for all NICUs.

Debbie Fraser, MN, RNC-NIC
Editor, *Neonatal Network: The Journal of Neonatal Nursing*

—◦◦◦—

Understanding the NICU is a breath of fresh air within the landscape of neonatal family educational resources. Zaichkin, Weiner, and Loren artfully weave together neonatal pathophysiology and management, family-centered care support, and real family experiences—making complex information tangible to the reader. This is an essential educational resource and supportive tool for anyone approaching or in the midst of a journey through the NICU.

Andrew C. Beckstrom, MD
Neonatologist, MEDNAX/Pediatrix Medical Group of Seattle

—◦◦◦—

Written with parents for parents, *Understanding the NICU* provides a summary of the realities that the emotional roller coaster of NICU care will bring, the victories that babies and families enjoy, and the outcomes that NICU babies and families can anticipate. Complete and nuanced, this book will help address questions, relieve anxiety, and inform parents during their baby's NICU stay.

F. Sessions Cole, MD
Park J. White, MD, Professor of Pediatrics and Director of the Division of Newborn Medicine, Washington University School of Medicine and St. Louis Children's Hospital

—◦◦◦—

—◦◦◦—

Understanding the NICU is a fantastic resource for NICU families. I love how it clearly explains so many NICU processes to parents who are immersed in that new environment. This book provides clear and vital information to families during a time of high stress with the birth of a premature or ill newborn. Every family will appreciate this book, both before and after delivery.

Marya Strand, MD, MS, FAAP
Associate Professor of Pediatrics, Saint Louis University School of Medicine;
Member, NRP Steering Committee

—◦◦◦—

Understanding the NICU: What Parents of Preemies and Other Hospitalized Newborns Need to Know is an essential go-to guide for all parents trying to navigate the complex, and sometimes overwhelming, world of the NICU. This easy-to-understand book has the perfect balance of reliable need-to-know medical information, helpful tips on navigating your baby's NICU stay, and hopeful stories of families "who have been there."

Unfamiliar terminology and complex NICU medical problems are simplified so parents can understand them, feel better prepared to communicate with their baby's care team, and participate in important decision-making.

Equally detailed attention is given to suggestions for successful parenting in the NICU environment.

But the standout feature of this book are the stories and pictures of real NICU babies and families interwoven with the medical information. These stories offer important encouragement and make the technical information more relatable.

A must-read for parents of NICU babies!

Linda McCarney, MSN, APRN, NNP-BC
Coordinator of NNP Education, Children's Hospital Colorado

—◦◦◦—

Reviewers

Susan W. Aucott, MD, FAAP

James J. Cummings, MD, FAAP

Beth Ellen Davis, MD, MPH, FAAP

Eric C. Eichenwald, MD, FAAP

Jay P. Goldsmith, MD, FAAP

Erin L. Keels, MS, APRN, NNP-BC

Lawrence M. Noble, MD, FAAP

Brenda Poindexter, MD, MS, FAAP

Karen M. Puopolo, MD, PhD, FAAP

Dan L. Stewart, MD, FAAP

Kristi Watterberg, MD, FAAP

To parents of babies who require newborn intensive care.
Find strength in knowledge. Face challenges with teamwork.
Celebrate each step forward.

Table of Contents

Family Story Icons

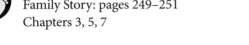

This page guides you to each family's personal photos, memories, and advice about parenting in the NICU. Find these family icons throughout the book and follow their unique journey as they provide guidance and support for your experience.

 Allison and **Reece,** 33 weeks
Family Story: pages 249–251
Chapters 3, 5, 7

 Kellan, 32 weeks
Family Story: pages 5–7
Chapters 1, 2, 5, 10

 August (Auggie), 24 weeks
Family Story: pages 77–80
Chapters 1, 3, 5, 6, 7, 8, 9, 10

 Lucy, 29 weeks
Family Story: pages 33–35
Chapters 1, 2, 3, 4, 5, 6, 7, 8, 9

 Bailey Jo and **Abraham,** 32 weeks 5 days
Family Story: pages 1–3
Chapters 2, 3, 5, 6, 8

 Maxwell, 34 weeks
Family Story: pages 161–163
Chapters 5, 8, 10

 Christopher, 32 weeks
Family Story: pages 9–11
Chapter 2

 Nathan, 24 weeks 4 days
Family Story: pages 53–55
Chapters 1, 4, 6, 7, 8, 9, 10

 Frankie, 29 weeks
Family Story: pages 133–135
Chapters 1, 2, 3, 5, 10

 Niklas, Gabbie, and **Lukas,** 28 weeks 4 days
Family Story: pages 219–221
Chapters 3, 6

 Holland and **Eden,** 24 weeks 3 days
Family Story: pages 103–106
Chapters 3, 4, 5, 6, 7, 8, 9, 10

 Pascal, 41 weeks 2 days
Family Story: pages 57–59
Chapters 2, 3, 4, 6, 8, 9

 Jack, 29 weeks, and **Henry,** 31 weeks
Family Story: pages 253–255
Chapters 3, 5, 8

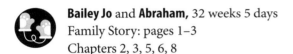 **Sienna,** 31 weeks 4 days
Family Story: pages 189–191
Chapters 3, 7

Please Note

· · · · · · · · · ·

We know that you would prefer to read "he" if your baby is a boy and "she" if your baby is a girl. It is difficult to communicate with the distraction of "his/her" and "he/she," however. Therefore, the baby's gender in this book varies by chapter.

Acknowledgments

Thanks to the American Academy of Pediatrics publishing staff, who believe in this book and its potential to help NICU parents navigate their journey.

Thank you to the many people who contributed to the photographs for this book.

Gigi O'Dea of Memory Portraits by Gigi, Sarasota, FL, for contributing several amazing photographs of NICU babies and their families, including the photo for our cover

Tamera Miller, RNC, NNP, at the University of Michigan

A special thank you to all of the parents who contributed stories and photos of their NICU experience and beyond. Your pictures are worth a thousand words.

Thank you to the health care professionals, whose unique contributions are much appreciated.

F. Sessions Cole, MD
St Louis Children's Hospital

Vicki E. Cronin, RN
Seattle Children's Hospital, Seattle, WA

Merllie Flores, RNC-OB, C-EFM
Swedish Medical Center, Seattle, WA

Debbie Fraser, MN, RNC-NIC
Athabasca University, Athabasca, Alberta, Canada

Susan Greenleaf, RNC-NIC, BSN
MultiCare Tacoma General Hospital, Tacoma, WA

Cynthia Jensen, RN, MS, CNS
University of California San Francisco Benioff Children's Hospital at Mission Bay, San Francisco, CA

Cheryl W. Major, RNC-NIC, BSN

Linda McCarney, MSN, APRN, NNP-BC
Children's Hospital Colorado, Aurora, CO

Sally Muskett, BSN, RNC-NIC, CPLC
University of Washington Medical Center, Seattle, WA

Michelle Walters, MN, RN
Swedish Medical Center, Seattle, WA

We wish to acknowledge these health care professionals, whose excellent work provided the foundation on which this book was created.

Julie M.R. Arafeh, RN, MSN

Debbie Fraser, MN, RNC-NIC

J. Craig Jackson, MD, MHA, FAAP

Patricia Jason, RN, BSN, CCRN

John Kattwinkel, MD, FAAP

Terrie Lockridge, MSN, RNC-NIC

Brenda Lee Lykins, ARNP

Denise Maguire, PhD, RN-BC, CNL

Lori A. Markham, MSN, MBA, NNP-BC, CCRN

Cindy C. Martin, MSN, RN, IBCLC, CKC

Karen Menghini, RN, MSN, NNP-BC

Lauren Thorngate, PhD, RN, CCRN

TrezMarie T. Zotkiewicz, RNC-NIC, MN, APRN

Introduction

The birth of a baby is one of the most personal, exhausting, beautiful, and emotionally charged events of a lifetime. But when everything does not go as expected—if labor is complicated or your baby is born preterm or facing serious complications—different emotions take over. If your baby is now in the neonatal intensive care unit (NICU), you may be feeling anxious, confused, guilty, angry, and even sad over the loss of the uncomplicated, healthy birth experience you had envisioned.

This book can help you understand the NICU and how you can best meet this challenge. It was written by professionals with decades of NICU experience in partnership with 14 families whose babies spent their first weeks, and sometimes months, in the NICU. Each family's story is unique, yet they all share common themes of strength and determination. Every parent was afraid, but they all learned to navigate the complex world of the NICU and become valuable members of their baby's health care team. You will learn, through their words, about the NICU parent experience—from birth, through intensive care, to homecoming, and beyond.

We invite you to become an important member of your baby's health care team. We believe parents can and should play an active role in their baby's care. This book was written for parents who want to learn about their baby's illness, how to overcome the barriers to parenting in the NICU, and how to nurture their NICU graduate at home.

You will not need all the information in this book because your baby will not have every problem described here. Look at the table of contents to find the sections that interest you most—and know that what interests you will change as your baby progresses through hospitalization. As you read through the sections that pertain to your baby, you may notice some parts of your baby's treatment are somewhat different than what is described here. That is because treatment approaches vary across the country and nursing and medical research is constantly changing the way babies in the NICU are managed. Ask your baby's team about any differences that concern you.

As you read the stories of families who volunteered to share their experiences, you will notice that some families have recent NICU experience, while others have NICU graduates who have already started school. All of these parents agreed to share their intensely personal stories so they could give you hope and help you discover your own strengths during hospitalization and as your child grows. A complete list of all the family stories is included on page xiii.

The NICU can be a place of remarkable healing. You will meet other parents whose support will give you strength. You will meet health care professionals who have devoted their careers to helping babies like yours. You will discover that the NICU offers a unique blend of technology and compassion that encourages healing and growth not only for babies, but also for parents. Learning to be a good parent never ends. We hope you get a good start here.

Jeanette Zaichkin, RN, MN, NNP-BC
Gary Weiner, MD, FAAP
David Loren, MD, FAAP

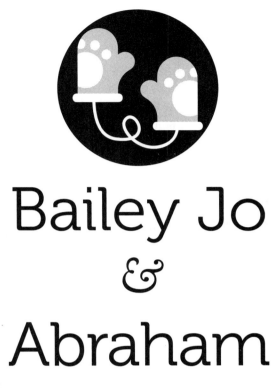

Bailey Jo
&
Abraham

Born at 32 weeks 5 days

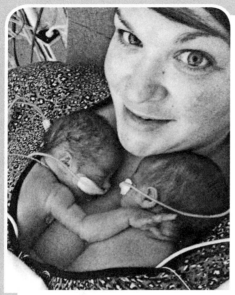

Mom cuddles Abraham and Bailey Jo.

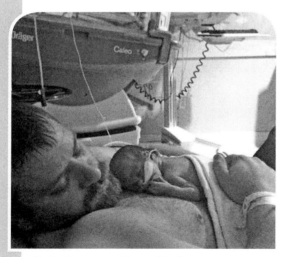

Dad enjoys some skin-to-skin time.

Bailey Jo and Abraham were born in 2014 at 32 weeks 5 days of gestation due to preeclampsia. I remember the first time I saw them—I had to wait until I was out of recovery from my cesarean. They were so tiny. Abraham weighed 4 pounds 1 ounce and Bailey Jo weighed 3 pounds 10 ounces. I wasn't allowed to hold them; I could stick my hand into the incubator and touch them. I remember crying and feeling so helpless.

Abraham was treated for mild respiratory distress and required nasal high-flow oxygen. Bailey Jo's respiratory distress was a little more of a concern and she was on a continuous positive airway pressure (CPAP) machine for the first 8 days until she was weaned to room air. Both were treated with phototherapy for jaundice. Both babies were also treated for apnea of prematurity, which was very scary. They would just stop breathing and an alarm would go off and nurses would run in, jiggle the babies a little, and then they would breathe again. That became normal for us, and it got to the point where the alarm would go off and by the time the nurses arrived, we had gotten them breathing. The twins also needed feeding support and had nasogastric (NG) tubes.

The first time I held them was so scary. They had all these tubes and cords and monitors hooked up to them. The nurses were so kind and not only caring for our tiny babies, but me as well. We live 60 miles away from the hospital; I stayed in special housing, which allowed me to be with the babies every day. My husband worked during the week and would come down every weekend, bringing our oldest, Lydia, who was 7 at the time. I would get up every morning and get to the hospital before rounds and leave after the shift change between 8:00 and 8:30 pm. I didn't want to miss anything. I remember one of the nurses telling me I had to eat and take a nap. She even went to the cafeteria and got me lunch. The nurses became like family. They listened, they loved our babies, and they were our biggest advocates.

Abraham was released after 24 days—completely off oxygen and taking 100% of his feeds by mouth. So we had one twin released and one still in the NICU. The NICU staff were so accommodating, letting me bring Abraham to the NICU with me every day to see Bailey Jo. It was hard being away from home and family. Finally, on day 34, we had our whole family home.

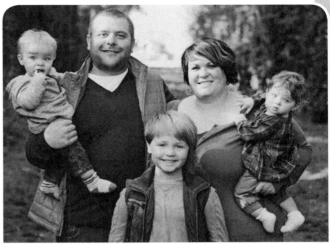

Bailey Jo and Abraham at 15 months of age with their parents and big sister, Lydia.

Now they are thriving 15-month-old toddlers with amazing little personalities. They love music and dancing, they adore their big sister, and she loves them just as much. They are growing and changing and learning every day. We have stayed in contact with several of our nurses and stop in for visits. I have never met a more caring and compassionate group of nurses and doctors. We could not have asked for a better experience in the NICU.

Bridget and Matthew, parents of Bailey Jo and Abraham

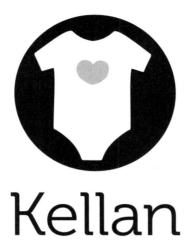

Kellan

Born at 32 weeks

In 2012, only hours after celebrating our little miracle at his baby shower, my water broke and contractions began. Kellan Patrick joined the world at 4 pounds 13 ounces, exactly 32 weeks' gestation.

The reality of what was happening did not kick in when the contractions did. It didn't even kick in when I delivered in the operating room and my son was whisked off. It was all so surreal and I was only thinking about the fact that I had gotten to meet the baby that I had waited for, for so long. What I had envisioned for those moments after birth was not at all what I experienced and it was hard to accept. I had to accept that other people were going to be responsible for helping my baby survive. The statement, "It will get worse before it gets better," became all too real, all too quickly.

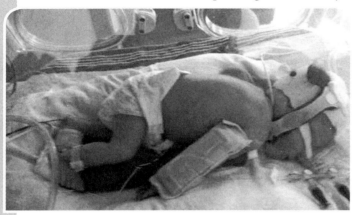

Kellan, at 32 weeks' gestation, resting on his tummy. CPAP is attached to his face with a special headgear, while an arm board keeps his IV in place at his side.

On his second day of life, Kellan was having trouble breathing on his own, so he was intubated. It was at that exact moment that I realized how serious this whole situation was. That moment defined me as a new mom of a preemie.

This photo was taken on Kellan's first birthday. I wanted to capture another side of the journey we had been on—the side that represented him home and growing. I want to always remember, and have him know, just how special he is and how far he has come.

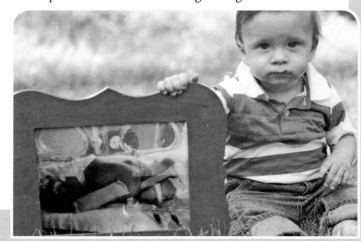

Kellan at age 1, with his NICU photo.

The following day, I was released from the hospital and had to cope with going home without my baby. In the days to follow, I was at his side from 9:00 am to 9:00 pm, participating in changing, feeding (even breastfeeding), kangarooing him, and being there to listen and learn during rounds. I was determined to take it all in and be as involved in his care and recovery as I could.

We did experience some delay in gross motor skills in the first 6 months, as well as speech delays at age 2, but we remained committed to making sure Kellan had the resources he needed to reach his milestones at his own pace. Although not accepted at 6 months of age, he was accepted into the Early On Program offered in our county and he received monthly visits from a speech therapist for 1 year.

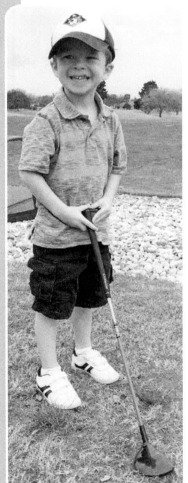

Today, Kellan is all boy and loves all things sports. He can tell you the name of all 32 NFL teams just by the look of their helmet and asks to hit balls at the golf range at every opportunity. The only thing bigger than his imagination is his heart, and he melts ours with his fun personality and his love for his little sister.

We had 37 days of ups and downs but a lifetime ahead of being grateful for the knowledge of the people around us. The dedication they had to helping Kellan survive! Our story could have been worse, and many are. We will never forget those who saved Kellan's life. They are the same people who taught us so much about the NICU journey as well as our journey as new parents.

Marnie, mother of Kellan

Kellan, at age 3.

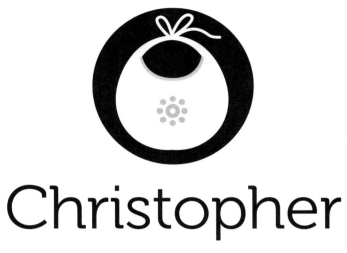

Christopher

Born at 32 weeks

My son, Christopher, was born 2 months premature in 2002. At birth, Christopher weighed in at 3 pounds 14 ounces and spent 28 days in the NICU.

I had lost a baby at 5 months' gestation and then had a miscarriage in the first trimester before Christopher was born. So when Christopher was born 8 weeks premature, I was scared and thought he was going to be taken from me too. I can remember when my husband and I went to see him one night and when we arrived, we were told that the doctor wanted to see us. Her first words were, "We've been trying to call you all day," and I lost it at that point. She asked me not to get upset and only wanted to tell us that Christopher's nurse had noticed that he was sleepier than normal, so they ran a bunch of tests and discovered he had an infection that is pretty common in preemies. So Christopher was on antibiotics for the next 10 days. We were constantly on an emotional roller coaster.

He came home on oxygen and an apnea monitor for another 2 months at home. He had follow-up appointments for the apnea and soon was taken off of the monitor and oxygen.

Christopher is now 13 years old and in the eighth grade. He is doing excellent in school academically. This is his fourth year in band. He plays the clarinet. Outside of the band, he is also in a jazz band taught by his band teacher. This is his third year doing that.

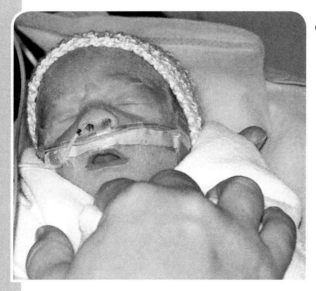

Christopher, at age 10 days.

When you have a child born too soon, you don't know what the outcome is going to be. You wonder if they are going to be like other children who were born healthy. Your life is different and I truly think it makes you a better person. If you weren't a strong person, you become one. That little person is depending on you.

Christine, mother of Christopher

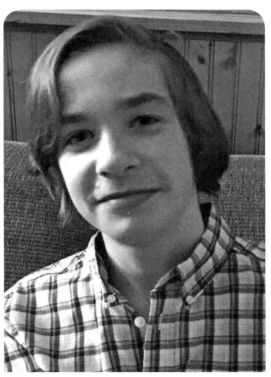

Christopher, at age 13.

An Unexpected Beginning

"The reality of what was happening did not kick in when the contractions did. It didn't even kick in when I delivered in the operating room and my son was whisked off. It was all so surreal and what I had envisioned for the moments after birth was not at all what I had experienced. That was hard to accept. Finally, the reality hit me and I had to accept the fact that other people were going to help my baby survive."

*Marnie, mother of **Kellan***

Giving birth is an adventure unlike any other life experience. Most parents anticipate the big event with a mixture of excitement and apprehension, yet few are truly prepared for any complications that may result in a baby needing intensive care.

Most of the time, the circumstances that result in a high-risk birth are beyond anyone's control. Even with the best prenatal care, a neonatal intensive care unit (NICU) admission is sometimes unavoidable. No one chooses a complicated pregnancy, an early delivery, or for their newborn to be admitted into the NICU. Finding out that pregnancy, labor, and birthing may pose risks to the mother's health or that your unborn baby may have health problems can be frightening. Understanding the basics of birthing "at risk" may help you cope with the stress that accompanies a different beginning.

Problems in Pregnancy That May Affect Your Baby

Babies develop within the complex environment of their mother's uterus. This is called the baby's *prenatal environment*. The fetus depends on its mother for oxygen and nutrition until birth, usually between about 39 and 41 weeks of pregnancy. This dependence means a mother's health and well-being are very important to her growing baby. Alcohol, drugs (including misuse of prescription drugs), and cigarettes create a risky environment for a growing fetus. In addition, some medical conditions and pregnancy complications can affect a developing fetus. The most commonly monitored conditions include

- Diabetes

- High blood pressure

- Infection

- Blood type incompatibilities

Diabetes and How It Might Affect Your Baby

When you eat, your pancreas secretes a hormone called *insulin* that keeps your blood sugar (*blood glucose*) levels within a healthy range. Diabetes happens when the body does not make enough insulin or does not use insulin properly. When this happens, blood glucose levels can be too high.

Some women already have diabetes before they become pregnant. Others are unable to produce enough insulin or their insulin does not work properly to control blood sugar levels when they become pregnant. This is a condition called *gestational diabetes*. In either case, the mother's blood glucose may rise to higher than normal levels. Extra glucose easily crosses into the developing fetus and the fetal pancreas responds by producing extra insulin. Increased glucose and insulin levels change the fetal environment and can harm the developing baby. If diabetes is present before conception, the baby's organs may not develop normally and there is an increased risk of serious birth defects (*congenital anomalies*). Higher than normal glucose and insulin levels later in pregnancy may cause the baby to have excess fat, breathing problems after birth, problems with low blood sugar after birth (*hypoglycemia*), and higher risks of obesity and diabetes later in life. For women with diabetes, their baby's health depends on keeping their blood glucose within a healthy range before conception and throughout their pregnancy.

High Blood Pressure and How It Might Affect Your Baby

Blood pressure does not usually increase during pregnancy, but high blood pressure does complicate about 6% to 8% of pregnancies in the United States.

- A woman who has high blood pressure before she becomes pregnant or develops high blood pressure before 20 weeks of gestation is said to have *chronic hypertension.*

- A woman who develops high blood pressure after 20 weeks of gestation is said to have *gestational hypertension.*

Some women with gestational hypertension go on to develop an additional complication of pregnancy known as *preeclampsia.* This occurs when, in addition to high blood pressure, there are signs other organs are not working normally. One common sign of preeclampsia is protein leaking from the kidneys into the urine. Women with chronic hypertension are more at risk for developing preeclampsia than women who do not have chronic hypertension. Preeclampsia may progress to more severe conditions, including *HELLP syndrome* and *eclampsia.* HELLP stands for *h*emolysis (breakdown of red blood cells), *e*levated *l*iver enzymes, and *l*ow *p*latelets. If a woman with preeclampsia develops seizures, the condition is called eclampsia. HELLP syndrome and eclampsia can be life-threatening conditions for the mother and fetus.

If a mother develops gestational hypertension, medications may be prescribed to lower her blood pressure. The doctor may recommend additional testing and will monitor the baby's growth for the remainder of her pregnancy. If her blood pressure stays high, blood flow to her kidneys, liver, brain, and uterus can be reduced. This can limit the baby's supply of oxygen and nutrients. The doctor may recommend early delivery if the mother develops severe high blood pressure that does not respond to treatment, if the mother shows signs of severe preeclampsia, or if her baby is showing signs of poor growth.

Infection During Pregnancy and How It Might Affect Your Baby

Infections during pregnancy that affect the developing fetus are most commonly caused by bacteria, viruses, or, very rarely, things like a fungus or a parasite. Although many infections that mothers can experience during pregnancy will resolve without causing any harm to the developing baby, some organisms can cross the placenta and cause a congenital infection that harms developing organs. Among the risks of maternal infection are preterm birth, miscarriage, abnormal fetal growth and development, abnormal blood cell counts, jaundice, seizures, and pneumonia. Many of these infections can be prevented by being up-to-date on immunizations before pregnancy and following good health practices to decrease exposure to infections. Even with good health care, some maternal infections cannot be prevented and may affect the baby. Common newborn infections are discussed in Chapter 4.

Blood Type Incompatibility and How It Might Affect Your Baby

All humans have substances attached to the surface of their red blood cells called blood group *antigens*. The specific combination of antigens determines your blood type, which is described by a series of letters and names, such as blood type A-positive. The most commonly discussed parts of your blood type are the ABO system and the Rh (positive or negative) system. Blood group antigens, and your blood type, are inherited, with a portion coming from each of your parents. If parents have more than one child, each child may inherit a unique combination of antigens and have a different blood type.

Your immune system protects your body from "foreign" cells by creating antibodies. If a baby's red blood cells have an antigen that the mother's blood lacks, the mother's immune system may identify the baby's blood as "foreign" and produce antibodies that cross the placenta and destroy fetal blood cells. These are called incompatible blood types. Most commonly, this happens if the mother is type O and the baby is type A or type B (*ABO incompatible*) or if the mother is Rh-negative and the baby is Rh-positive (*Rh incompatible*). Rh incompatibility usually does not affect an Rh-negative woman's first pregnancy because her immune system has not been sensitized yet. ABO incompatibility may affect a type-O mother's first pregnancy because type-O mothers often have anti-A and anti-B antibodies even without exposure to fetal blood. In addition to the ABO and Rh groups, red blood cells have other "minor" antigens that may cause incompatibility.

Blood group incompatibilities can cause the fetus to have a low red blood cell count (become *anemic*). Usually, ABO incompatibility causes milder disease than Rh incompatibility. Severe anemia occurs in only about 1% of all ABO-incompatible pregnancies. But if the mother's antibody response against her fetus is very strong, as is often the case with Rh incompatibility, red blood cell destruction may cause severe anemia before birth. High-risk pregnancies with known blood group incompatibilities are followed by ultrasound for signs of severe anemia. Sometimes, the fetus will develop swelling and signs of heart failure (*fetal hydrops*) and will need to receive blood transfusions before birth.

Because Rh incompatibility is preventable and causes serious complications for the fetus and newborn, mothers who are Rh-negative are followed very closely throughout their pregnancies. Rh-negative mothers usually receive a medication called *RhoGAM* (*WinRho* in Canada) at the beginning of the third trimester and after any procedure that causes fetal blood to cross into the mother's bloodstream. RhoGAM may block the mother's immune system from producing antibodies against fetal red blood cells, but it is effective only for women who have not already formed these antibodies.

Fetal Factors That Affect Your Baby

Gestational Age

Gestational age is the number of completed weeks that have elapsed between the first day of the mother's last menstrual period and the current date. By asking, "What is the baby's gestational age?" the care provider can determine if the baby is term, preterm, or post-term. Gestational age is correlated with birth weight, length, and measurement of the head to categorize the baby's size as appropriate for gestational age (*AGA*), small for gestational age (*SGA*), or large for gestational age (*LGA*).

What Is Gestational Age?

Gestational age, which is the time from the last menstrual period until birth, determines whether a newborn is term (on time) or preterm (born early). In simple terms, a baby born before 37 weeks' gestation is preterm; however, gestational ages can be described in the following periods:

- **Extremely preterm:** born at or before 25 weeks of pregnancy
- **Very preterm:** born at less than 32 weeks of pregnancy
- **Moderately preterm:** born between 32 and 34 weeks of pregnancy
- **Late preterm:** born between 34 and 36 weeks of pregnancy
- **Early term:** born between 37 and 39 weeks of pregnancy
- **Full term:** born between 39 and 41 weeks of pregnancy
- **Late term:** born between 41 and 42 weeks of pregnancy
- **Post-term (also called postdates):** born after 42 weeks of pregnancy

Gestational age is usually determined by the date of the woman's last menstrual period. However, this date may be uncertain. Ultrasound in the first trimester of pregnancy is accurate for predicting the due date within 3 to 5 days. After that, ultrasound estimates a due date within 1 or 2 weeks.

Multiple-Gestation Pregnancies

If there is more than one baby (called a *multiple-gestation pregnancy*), lack of space in the uterus can affect one or more baby's weight gain during the final third of pregnancy. Through week 29 of a healthy pregnancy, the growth rates of multiple fetuses are nearly the same as for one. But at 30 weeks of gestation and later, multiple fetuses do not gain weight as rapidly as a single fetus does.

A second risk for more than one fetus is abnormal blood flow through the placenta. If your babies came from a single egg, the fetuses are called *identical* and usually share one placenta (*monochorionic*). If your babies came from more than one egg, the fetuses are *not identical* and each has its own placenta (*dichorionic*). Identical twins frequently have connections between the blood vessels in their shared placenta that can cause abnormal blood flow patterns between the twins. This is called a *twin-to-twin transfusion.* One twin receives too much blood, while the other receives too little. The twin who gets less blood flow (the donor twin) can show signs of poor growth, anemia, poor kidney function, and heart failure. The twin who receives too much blood (the recipient) is often sicker and can also show signs of heart failure.

Women with multiple-gestation pregnancies are also at higher risk of developing gestational diabetes, gestational hypertension, preeclampsia, and preterm birth.

Congenital Anomalies (Birth Defects)

Because ultrasound during pregnancy is so common, physical abnormalities in a baby may be detected before birth.

The medical term for these variations is *congenital* (meaning "existing at birth") *anomalies,* and they may also be called *birth defects.* Congenital anomalies may appear as a single finding, or there may be several together. While many congenital anomalies discovered by prenatal ultrasound are minor and not expected to cause any significant problem, some congenital anomalies are significant and may cause serious or even life-threatening problems after birth, and some will have unknown significance and an uncertain effect on the baby until after the birth. It is important to note that not all congenital anomalies can be detected by ultrasound.

When a congenital anomaly is discovered before the baby's birth, parents and their health care team usually have time to discuss the findings, meet with additional experts, obtain additional tests, and prepare in advance for any special needs.

When congenital anomalies are found in a baby before birth, parents are often referred to a specialized team of experts composed of providers for mom (maternal-fetal medicine specialists) and baby (for example, neonatologists, genetics experts, surgeons, pediatric subspecialists such as cardiologists or neurologists, developmental pediatricians). These teams work together in a prenatal diagnosis center or clinic. If a congenital anomaly has been found in your baby, you will learn much more about what this means and what can be done about it from this team of experts. These teams will often show you pictures, videos, or models to help you understand what is happening to your baby. They may also help you connect with other parents whose baby had similar problems. Many congenital anomalies or diseases have treatments that are still being developed, so you may discover that not all NICUs or specialist teams will manage a problem the same way.

Many parents want more information and will look for additional details, advice, and stories from other parents on the Internet and social media. However, research has consistently shown that the Web contains plenty of inaccurate medical information, and social media sites can also have misleading or biased medical information. Ask your medical team for recommended sources of reliable information.

Where Will You Give Birth?

Your baby's health may depend on decisions made before his birth. By working with your team of doctors, nurses, nurse practitioners, midwives, and other health care professionals in making these decisions, you are acting as a responsible parent even before your baby is born. Your team's first recommendation may concern the hospital where your baby will be born.

When Your Baby Needs Surgery

When you first hear the words, "Your baby might need surgery," you may be overwhelmed by questions. For most parents, the most common questions are, "Who will be involved?"; "What will the surgery involve?"; "Will my baby be all right?"; and, "What can I do to help?"

Not all hospitals have the experts to do neonatal surgery. If your baby needs a special type of surgery, such as heart surgery, you may be referred to a large university medical center or a children's hospital. Transfer to another hospital, especially if it is far from your home, may present more challenges, such as transportation, more time off from work, and child care for your other children. Your baby's social worker or care coordinator can help you navigate the system and decrease some of your stress.

Levels of Care

Your hospital's designated level of maternal and neonatal care may affect where your baby is born. Although every hospital is equipped to handle emergencies, many smaller community hospitals prefer to transport high-risk women and babies to a larger medical center where staff are more experienced at managing complicated pregnancies and sick newborns.

The American Academy of Pediatrics has proposed standard definitions for neonatal levels of care (levels I through IV). Interpretation and application of these levels vary across the United States, but a higher level of care means there are more intensive care specialists and services available for your newborn. If your care team determines that your labor or your baby's birth may become complicated, its best recommendation may be that you be transported to a hospital that offers a higher level of care before your baby is born.

> The whole experience was surreal and overwhelming. We simply didn't know what to expect from a baby born 2½ months early, and we weren't prepped, mentally or logistically, for her arrival.
>
> Matthew, father of **Lucy**

Maternal Transport: What Can You Expect?

If your baby is expected to require specialized care and you are at a hospital that does not offer these services, transporting the expectant mother (*maternal transport*) may be a good idea so your newborn can be admitted directly into the NICU. If your baby is born in a community hospital that does not provide neonatal intensive care, your newborn may need to be transported after birth, which can be stressful and separate you and your baby. Maternal transport is not possible if the expectant mother is so seriously ill that transport would further endanger her health or safety or if labor has progressed to the point where birth could happen during transport. In these cases, it is safer to give birth at the community hospital and stabilize the newborn for transport.

Even though maternal transport may be necessary to get the care your baby needs, it will change some of your plans. When you change hospitals, you may not have your own doctor or midwife to deliver your baby and your regular pediatrician may not be directly involved in your baby's care. You may be far from home, without the support of family and friends. Maternal transport may mean making long-term arrangements to care for your household and other children. Your family may worry about the mother's health and the uncertain health of your baby. Transport can feel like an emergency, and the nonpregnant parent may feel all the responsibility for holding things together.

During this stressful time, partners need to communicate honestly with each other, support each other, and be together, if possible, when information is given. Stress can make it difficult to understand everything you're told. If you and your partner hear the information together, you may be able to better clarify the facts for one another.

The staff at the community hospital or a member of the transport team should provide you with directions to the medical center and its perinatal unit. Your case manager or the hospital social worker should be able to tell you about affordable lodging and parking discounts at or near the medical center. He or she can also provide other important information to help you navigate an unfamiliar place.

Your Care Providers

The people attending your baby's birth will depend on your circumstances. When the mother is sick or labor becomes complicated, many interventions become necessary and people with equipment rapidly fill the room.

The following list describes the care providers you may encounter during labor. Chapter 2 is devoted to helping you understand the roles of people in the NICU.

Labor Nurses

Your labor nurses are important sources of information, serve as your advocates, and provide links to the other people involved in the process of labor and birth.

Physicians

Several different physicians may be involved in your hospital care, including obstetricians (specialists in pregnancy, labor, and delivery), perinatologists (specialists in high-risk maternal and fetal medical care), anesthesiologists (specialists in pain management), and neonatologists (specialists in newborn intensive care). In a teaching hospital, students and physicians in training (including medical students, residents, and fellows) may also be involved.

Other Hospital Personnel

In addition to your labor nurses and physicians, you may meet other specialized hospital staff. Laboratory personnel may draw blood samples; a sonographer may perform an ultrasound; and a social worker may meet with you to discuss available resources and your personal and family needs. Each member of the team provides an important aspect of hospital care.

Questions to Ask About the Plan of Care

You may have many questions about the plan of care, but because of the stressful situation, you may have difficulty remembering all of your questions. It may help to keep a journal and write down all of your questions as they come to mind. Keep it with you at all times. Some questions you may have for your team include

- How long is this hospital stay? Is hospital discharge possible before the baby is born?
- What activities are permitted? Using the restroom and shower? Or does "bed rest" mean staying in bed all the time?
- Is a regular diet served during this hospitalization or is there a special diet?
- What signs and symptoms should be reported to the nurse or doctor?
- Why might an emergency birth be necessary?
- If an emergency birth is necessary, what will happen? Who can attend the birth as the support person?

When you are nervous, it is normal to forget what you are told and not hear all of the information you are given. Write down the answers to your questions in your journal so you can refer to them later. If you have more questions or have forgotten the answers, you may always ask questions again. The health care team wants you to be as comfortable as possible in this situation.

What to Expect From the Team

In general, you should expect courteous and respectful treatment at all times. All members of your health care team should introduce themselves by name and job title before performing examinations or asking questions. Even in an emergency, team members should protect your privacy by closing hallway doors and using privacy screens during caregiving. Communication may not be easy for you at this difficult time, but keep in mind that you are an important part of the team and your input is valuable.

Obstetric Care Plans

Talking with the obstetric team and asking questions will give you vital information about the care plan. Discussing this information with your partner or others you trust will help you and your health care team make the best decisions for your baby and your family.

Finding a New Plan

If you have reached the point in your pregnancy when you have planned your labor and birth experience but then find you are at risk, you may still be able to keep part of your plan. If your physician recommends a cesarean birth, for example, ask if you may play the music you planned for labor in the operating room. Having some control over your care may reduce the intensity of your feelings of loss for the "perfect" birth and may help resolve some of your emotions.

Corticosteroids

If there is a strong chance your baby will be born very preterm, your doctor may recommend that the mother receive *corticosteroids* (often referred to simply as *steroids*). Steroids have several important benefits for preterm newborns, including decreasing the severity of breathing problems, improving blood pressure, and decreasing the chance of bleeding in the brain. Steroids work best about 48 hours after the first dose and continue to work for about 7 days. This single course of steroid therapy given to the mother is safe and does not hurt the baby's growth or development.

> "My team of doctors did everything they could to try and stop the labor from progressing. Within hours, they determined that our little man was coming whether we were ready or not. Our doctor came in and started going over what we could expect...what they were hoping for but also what they were hoping would not happen."
>
> Marnie, mother of **Kellan**

Vaginal or Cesarean Birth?

When spontaneous vaginal birth is safe for the mother and baby, this is usually the option of choice. Vaginal birth eliminates the risks of surgical complications and shortens the mother's hospital stay and recovery period.

Any condition that causes concern about the baby's well-being, such as trouble with the fetal heart rate or serious bleeding or illness, may make cesarean birth the best choice for a healthy outcome. Other common reasons for cesarean birth include previous cesarean births, failure to make progress in labor, and unusual fetal presentation (for example, the baby is not positioned to deliver headfirst). The experience and training your caregivers have in this type of medical and nursing care will guide their clinical judgment. The information they give you is based on careful consideration of the risks and benefits of each birthing method.

If preterm labor cannot be stopped and a vaginal birth is expected, you may discover that labor and birth progress quickly. Even though vaginal birth is a natural process, an unusually fast birth (a *precipitous birth*) can be frightening. Because caregivers and equipment must move quickly, a precipitous birth often feels like an emergency. Your doctor and labor nurse will support you through the urgency of the birth. Afterward, ask them to help you review what happened and clarify details that are important to you.

A Difficult Question: "Will My Baby Live?"

"Will my baby live?" is a common question asked by parents who face a high-risk birth. This is a difficult question, and the answer depends on many factors.

If there's time before the birth, your obstetric provider and the neonatologist or pediatrician will speak with you about what to expect when your baby is born. As your baby's parent, you are expected to help make health care decisions in your baby's best interests. In most situations, you will be asked to participate in the choices and decisions that affect your baby's care at birth. If birth is about to happen or has become an emergency, it may be difficult to get all of the information you need and have time to think about your choices. This makes clear and ongoing communication with the neonatal team most important, so you can be kept updated on your baby's condition.

If your baby is expected to be extremely preterm, generally between 22 and 24 weeks of gestation, or if your baby is known to have a serious congenital anomaly, your health care professionals may talk with you and your partner about your baby's chances for survival and significant complications. This helps you share in the decision-making about what kind of medical care your baby will receive during the first minutes after birth. You may have the opportunity to discuss what, if any, limits you want to consider concerning resuscitation of your baby after birth. Every situation is unique and, sometimes, life-prolonging measures might cause suffering without resulting in any meaningful hope for recovery. In these cases, many parents simply want to hold and comfort their baby soon after birth. You may prefer something in between, such as beginning resuscitation by providing breathing assistance and then, depending on the baby's response and the advice of the medical provider, deciding to go ahead with more complex steps or stop and provide comfort only. It is important to know that resuscitation can be stopped after it starts, but it is not acceptable to provide comfort care only and then change the plan and start resuscitation many minutes after the baby is born. A baby who survives a delayed resuscitation is at risk of serious disability.

> ❝ I was only 24 weeks' pregnant. There was nothing I could say or do to change what was about to happen. My body had failed my child. Only later would I understand this feeling of guilt more fully. There was so much more we were about to learn, about our son, about ourselves, about the exhausting and complicated journey of a baby born much too soon, about love that is deferred. ❞
>
> Robyn, mother of **Auggie**

Your NICU team cannot make any promises about what will happen after the delivery. If the baby's condition at birth is different than expected, the plan may change. In this case, the NICU team will keep you informed about your baby's condition and may offer some choices about next steps. Sometimes, resuscitating and admitting the baby to the NICU gives you and the medical team more time to gather information about the best plan of action and gives you more time to ask important questions.

What Can Happen at Birth

Occasionally, a baby is born sick without warning. Most of the time, the obstetric and neonatal team of doctors, nurses, and respiratory care practitioners anticipate problems and are ready to deal with them.

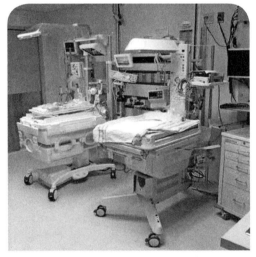

At every birth, members of the neonatal team work together to assess the baby's condition.

Every hospital and birthing center delivery area is equipped to provide lifesaving support to newborns. Resuscitation may take place in the delivery room or in a room nearby. In any case, preparing for the birth of a sick or preterm newborn brings tension into the room. A physician or a nurse practitioner usually leads the neonatal resuscitation team, and you may hear the team leader assigning duties and checking equipment. Caregivers are ready to help the newborn breathe and achieve or maintain the pulse and blood pressure necessary for life.

In many settings, the newborn receives lifesaving care in the delivery room. In other settings, a nearby room is used for evaluation and resuscitation, as pictured here.

> 66 We knew it would be an emergency C-section. The labor and delivery staff prepared me with everything I needed to know. Afterwards, they wheeled me into the NICU on a stretcher. The nurses and doctors were connecting **Frankie** to all her monitors. I honestly believe I was in complete shock. I didn't hear a word they were saying. 99
>
> Lisa, mother of **Frankie**

Resuscitation Activities

The steps taken to resuscitate a newborn depend on the baby's condition at birth and special needs.

First Steps

When your baby is born, the obstetric care providers may cover him with a warm towel and suction fluids out of his mouth and nose so he can breathe. If he is vigorous, they may wait 30 to 60 seconds to clamp and cut the umbilical cord. As long as the placenta is working as it should, this short delay allows a significant amount of additional blood to flow into the newborn after birth.

After the umbilical cord is clamped and cut, the baby may be moved to the radiant warmer, which is a portable cart with a mattress and a heat source overhead. Most babies are quickly wiped dry to prevent chilling; however, preterm babies less than 32 weeks' gestation are placed on the radiant warmer on top of a heating pad, covered with clear plastic wrap from the neck down, and wear a soft cloth hat to help prevent heat loss.

Breathing

Most babies make some crying efforts in the first minute after birth. The neonatal team may encourage breathing by gently rubbing the baby's back. If your baby does not breathe in a few moments, is too weak to breathe regularly, or has a slow pulse (*heart rate*), the neonatal team will place a soft mask over the baby's nose and mouth and use a mechanical device to inflate his lungs and assist his breathing. This is called *positive-pressure ventilation* (*PPV*). Most babies will respond with an increasing heart rate, and most will begin breathing on their own.

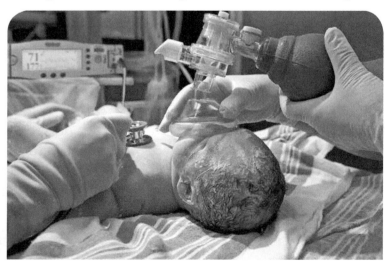

The caregiver places the face mask of the resuscitation bag firmly over the baby's nose and mouth and delivers air/oxygen into his lungs. Positive-pressure ventilation is necessary when the baby is not breathing or when his heart rate is slow.

Courtesy of Gigi O'Dea.

If your baby is breathing with a normal heart rate but appears to be struggling, the team may place a soft mask over his mouth and nose and use the device to hold a steady stream of air pressure in his lungs. This constant air pressure is called *continuous positive airway pressure* (*CPAP*) and helps to keep the baby's tiny air sacs in the lungs (*alveoli*) open between breaths. This makes breathing easier for the baby. Continuous positive airway pressure can also be given using tubing with short prongs that fit into the baby's nose or a special mask placed over the baby's nose. You may notice a bubbling bottle of water at the end of the tubing that supplies the air pressure.

Oxygen

The air we breathe (called room air) contains about 21% oxygen. During resuscitation, your baby's need for additional oxygen is monitored with *pulse oximetry*. A *pulse oximeter* is a device that wraps around the baby's hand or wrist to measure the amount of oxygen attached to his red blood cells. The device shines a small red light through the skin and is painless. The pulse oximeter

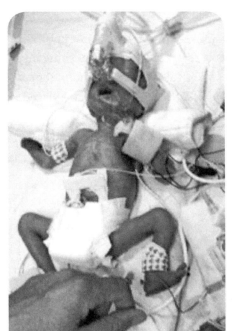

displays a number called *oxygen saturation* (abbreviated as SpO_2). Based on your baby's age in minutes, a special chart is used to identify his oxygen saturation "target" and guide the administration of additional oxygen.

Intubation

If your baby does not begin to breathe after several minutes of PPV or if his heart rate remains low, a thin plastic tube may be placed in his mouth and advanced into his windpipe (*trachea*). This process is called *intubation,* and the tube is called an *endotracheal tube.* An endotracheal tube provides a direct route to your baby's lungs and allows the team to help him breathe more effectively. The tube can be attached to a resuscitation device that temporarily provides additional air pressure and oxygen or to a respirator (*ventilator*) for more prolonged assistance with breathing. Because the tube is positioned between your baby's vocal cords, he will not be able to make crying noises while the tube is in place. When your baby no longer needs the endotracheal tube, it is removed. This is called *extubation.*

At 29 weeks of gestation, **Frankie** is doing her own breathing with CPAP, secured to her face with a special headgear. She has a "bridge" of white tape on her abdomen to secure her umbilical catheter.

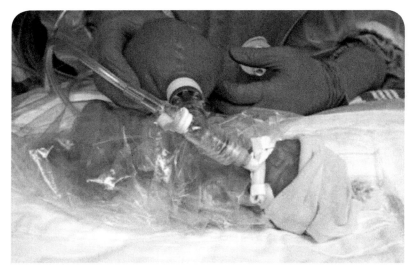

This is **Auggie** at 24 weeks of gestation and just minutes old. He wears a soft cloth hat and is wrapped in plastic to maintain his body temperature. The care provider holds the inflated bag and delivers gentle breaths into his lungs through his endotracheal tube.

Emergency Umbilical Venous Catheter

In rare cases, a baby is so seriously ill that his heart rate remains very low and does not improve with PPV through an endotracheal tube. When this happens, *chest compressions* (pushing on the baby's chest) and a lifesaving medication called *epinephrine* (also called *adrenaline*) may be needed. A thin tube called an emergency *umbilical venous catheter* (*UVC*) can be placed quickly into the large vein in the umbilical cord, allowing the neonatal team to give medications and fluids directly into the baby's bloodstream. A UVC may also be placed after resuscitation, if your baby needs an IV for more than a few days (see Chapter 3).

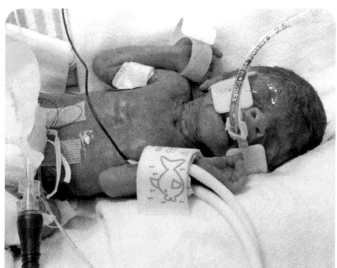

Nathan is 24 weeks' gestation and also required endotracheal intubation at his birth. Notice the tape and tubing on his abdomen where his umbilical catheter is secured. He has a blood pressure cuff on his left arm and instead of cardiac monitor leads that stick to his chest, he has limb leads. You can see one of the limb leads on his right upper arm.

Apgar Score

At 1 minute of age, again at 5 minutes, and every 5 minutes during resuscitation, your baby is assessed and given a number score to reflect his general condition. This scoring system was created by a physician, Dr Virginia Apgar, in the 1950s and is named after her. *Apgar scores* give the neonatal team an indication of your baby's overall condition and his transition to life outside of the womb. The score helps to standardize the way health care professionals describe a baby's transition. The Apgar score does not predict your baby's IQ or future intelligence.

To determine your baby's Apgar score, his health care team assesses 5 categories: heart rate, breathing, color, muscle tone, and reflexes. Babies are assigned a score of 0, 1, or 2 in each category, with 0 indicating absent or very depressed responses and 2 indicating very active responses. The Apgar score is the total of the 5 numbers. When the baby receives assistance at birth, an expanded Apgar score may be used (see the Expanded Apgar Score chart in the Appendix) to document what kind of help the baby was receiving when the score was assigned in each category.

Few babies receive an Apgar score of 10 because a baby's hands and feet normally remain blue for a while. A full-term, healthy, crying baby usually receives an Apgar score of 8 or 9. Keep in mind, however, that very preterm babies receive lower Apgar scores than full-term newborns simply because they are immature and unable to respond with loud crying and strong muscle tone.

Surfactant

Surfactant is a soapy substance normally produced by lung cells that helps to keep the lungs inflated. Production of surfactant begins at about 24 weeks of gestation but is not well developed until about 36 weeks of gestation. Some preterm babies will have breathing difficulty because they do not have enough surfactant in their lungs. Giving steroids to the mother before the birth (*antenatal steroids*) speeds up the production of surfactant in the baby's lungs. Many preterm newborns will improve by receiving breathing support with CPAP, but others will need to receive additional surfactant after birth. Surfactant can be instilled into the baby's lungs through an endotracheal tube.

If your baby will be born preterm, ask the neonatologist what you can expect with the use of CPAP and surfactant administration in the delivery room or NICU. (See Chapter 5.)

Newborn Transport to Another Hospital

If your baby requires additional specialized care that is not offered at your baby's birth hospital, he will be transported to a NICU at another hospital. Your baby's physician or nurse practitioner will arrange the transport. Depending on the condition of your baby and the distance between the baby's birth hospital and the NICU, your baby may be transported by ambulance, helicopter, or aircraft.

Newborn Transport Preparation

A specially trained neonatal transport team will prepare your baby for the trip and continue intensive care while traveling to the NICU. Your baby will be inside a transport incubator, designed to provide warmth while allowing immediate access for any care he may need during transport.

Immediately before your baby leaves the hospital, the transport team will bring the baby to the mother's bedside, if possible. Separation from your new baby is difficult. If the mother is still recovering from surgery, she may not even remember seeing the baby before transport. Some families take photos using their phone or camera before the baby leaves. Even if your baby is not critically ill, separation is frightening and increases your stress.

Before the transport team leaves, be sure you have the NICU phone number, know how you will be informed when your baby arrives at the NICU, and know how to call the NICU so that you can check on your baby whenever you wish.

> 66 A stay in the NICU is going to be temporary. They won't let you stay there forever even on those days when it really feels like you will be there forever. While it is difficult to not constantly look for the finish line (and everyone will ask, "When is the baby coming home?"), try to take it day by day and minute by minute and find happiness and joy in the experience. The NICU is an amazing place when you stop and look around. 99
>
> Kate, mother of **Lucy**

Staying in Touch

A member of your baby's care team at the receiving hospital will typically call you after your baby arrives at the NICU and update you on your baby's condition. If you do not understand what you are told, ask the NICU provider to explain the situation in words you can understand. The doctor and nurse at your birth hospital may also help explain your baby's condition.

If the NICU is far from the hospital, you and your partner may be faced with the additional challenge of figuring out how to be in 2 places at once. Long-distance transport is especially difficult if you have other children at home who need your attention.

Ask your hospital discharge planner or social worker about hotels near your baby, and try to spend some time with your baby as soon as possible. If you must return home right away, ask about the system for staying in touch with the NICU. Your baby's NICU doctor or nurse may set up a time to call you every day and tell you about your baby's progress, and you will be given the phone number to call whenever you wish. Some NICUs will send or e-mail you a photograph and short note "from your baby" each week. Some NICUs have a video system so you can see your baby on your laptop, tablet, or smartphone.

Sorting It Out

To process and understand their birthing experience, many new parents feel the need to tell and retell the story of labor and birth. This recounting of events can be especially important for parents of a baby who needs intensive care. When your baby's birth becomes a series of unexpected events, the whole experience may take on a dreamlike quality, making it hard for you to know what actually happened. Until the experience becomes real to you, coping with the challenges of NICU parenting can be difficult.

Each parent may have a slightly different version of what happened and feel varying levels of responsibility and powerlessness. Parents of babies in the NICU may feel a sense of loss and failure. They may feel torn in multiple directions trying to meet the needs of their other children, family members, sick newborn (or newborns), and partner. The NICU staff can be a great help as you search for answers to your questions and sort out your feelings. Once you begin to understand what happened and can place the events in order, you can begin to move ahead. This will not happen all at once or at the same time for everyone. Allow yourself time for personal recovery and take advantage of supportive people who will listen to your story. You will also discover that NICU parents often find support by sharing their experiences with other NICU parents. Your ability to cope will grow over time as you learn about the resources available and gain the strength to move forward.

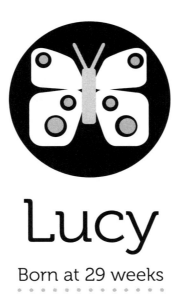

Lucy

Born at 29 weeks

I was just entering my third trimester and my pregnancy had gone relatively smoothly. I had a little bit of spotting over the weekend at 29 weeks and went to the hospital and checked out fine. Matt and I went to our routine prenatal appointment the next morning and I again checked out fine and was cleared to fly on a business trip the next day.

Matt and I said good-bye and I went to work. About 30 minutes later, my water broke. A friend drove me to the hospital and Matt met me there. They tried to slow things down, but Lucy had other ideas and was born at 5:39 that night. During her birth, Lucy's heart rate dropped dramatically and I was scared that we were going to lose her. It was overwhelming. She was 3 pounds 13 ounces and had a head full of hair. She was absolutely perfect.

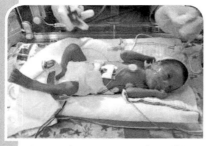
Lucy makes progress in the NICU.

During our NICU stay, Lucy had a lot of trouble with "events" (apnea and bradycardia), particularly with any attempts at feeding. She could not handle breastfeeding and struggled with bottles until right before our discharge day. It took us a few weeks to settle into a NICU routine, but once we found our rhythm and schedule, things became a lot easier and fun at times. The NICU is full of amazing people who dedicate their lives to treating and helping the tiniest of humans.

Our NICU stay was 71 days and we went home 3 days before my due date. Any NICU stay, no matter if it is a few hours or several months, is difficult and scary for parents. It is usually not part of your plan or what you envision for the start of your child's life and it is a surreal place that most people know very little about. Also, in the beginning, I struggled with a lot of guilt about why she came early and blamed myself for her early birth and struggles in the NICU.

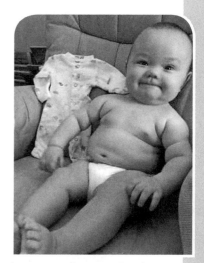
Lucy next to her preemie pajamas.

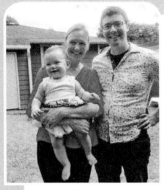

Lucy with her parents.

It is often hard to believe this girl was the little 3-pound preemie we fell in love with! Today, Lucy is toddling around our house, laughing and smiling and carrying on. It is so fun seeing her learn things on a daily basis and her vocabulary (both verbal and sign language) is exploding right now. In the last couple weeks, she's started nodding "yes" to things. She's become obsessed with cats (pictures of cats, actual cats, drawings of cats, even abstract illustrations of cats), which is particularly odd since we don't have a cat. Lucy also loves watermelon, books, baths, opening and closing everything, and all music.

Lucy is caring, gentle, and shy. In short, she's a fun little person, and she's awesome to spend time with. Looking back, I love that we got to know her when she was so little and got to see how she has grown and overcome so much since that day we met her.

Kate and Matthew, parents of Lucy

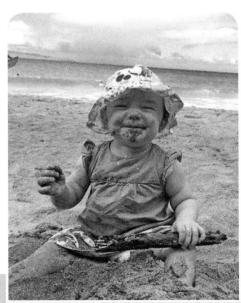

Lucy on the beach.

The NICU Journey Begins

> "When your child is born too soon, you don't know what the outcome is going to be. You wonder if they are going to be like other children who were born healthy. Your life is different, and I truly think it makes you a better person. If you weren't a strong person, you become one."
>
> *Christine, mother of **Christopher***

The moment of birth is usually a triumphant celebration. Not only have you made it through labor and birth, you've welcomed into your family a new little person who carries your dreams for the future. When things don't go as expected, you face a more stressful beginning than most parents. You and your partner need to deal with the feelings of loss that accompany the birth of a sick or preterm baby. For most parents, the neonatal intensive care unit (NICU) is a new world of medical vocabulary and technology that may, at first, seem overwhelming.

First Steps

Each neonatal intensive care nursery has its own routines, but most share certain common priorities when a new baby is admitted. Here are explanations of typical activities during NICU admission.

The Admission Process

When your baby enters the NICU, many things happen at once. Doctors, nurses, and respiratory care practitioners will stabilize your baby; begin diagnostic tests, if necessary; and plan her immediate care. Priorities in the first hour include making sure your baby is breathing well and keeping her oxygen saturation, heart rate, blood pressure, blood sugar, and body temperature all within normal levels. Your baby is weighed, a hospital identification bracelet is placed on her wrist or foot, she receives an injection of vitamin K to prevent potential bleeding difficulties, and antibiotic ointment is placed in her eyes to prevent infection. During the first hour, the NICU team may perform special procedures to assist your baby's breathing, obtain blood samples for tests, and insert thin tubes (*catheters*) into veins or arteries to give medications and fluids. While the team is performing these procedures, she may be under sterile drapes and you may need to wait to see her. Additional routine procedures, such as measuring her length and obtaining footprints, may be delayed until she is more stable.

First Trip to the NICU

Your NICU team will be very busy during the first hour of your baby's arrival. If you must wait to see her, minutes may seem like hours. Within the first 60 minutes, a member of the team should be available to give you and your partner an update, describe what procedures have been completed, and explain the initial plan. The team members will do everything they can to bring you to her bedside as quickly as possible and give you a chance to touch her, talk to her, and take photos.

The experience of becoming a NICU parent is different for everyone. Parents often describe their first day or two in the NICU as "foggy and dreamlike." You may feel helpless and wonder how you will ever be able to participate in your baby's care, especially if your baby is transported to the NICU from another hospital. Most NICU nurses and physicians are good at keeping parents informed. They will probably tell you more than you can understand at first, so don't worry if things seem unclear. Very soon, you will begin to understand your newborn's problems, get to know your NICU team, understand their routines, and begin to participate as partners in your baby's care.

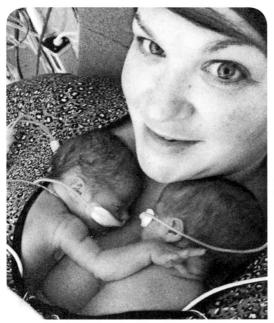

"The first time I held them was so scary. They had all these tubes and cords and monitors hooked up to them."

*Bridget, mother of **Bailey Jo** and **Abraham***

When you and your partner first arrive in the NICU, and every time you come after that, you will stop at a sink and wash your hands thoroughly. Depending on the NICU infection control policy, the staff may also have an alcohol hand-gel sanitizer at your baby's bedside and ask you to use it every time before and after you touch your baby.

Special Considerations for Moms

Depending on your baby's condition at birth, she may have been taken immediately to the NICU, without you getting as much as a glimpse of this new member of your family. If you experienced a high-risk birth or emergency cesarean delivery, you may have had general anesthesia and your partner or support person may not have been able to attend the birth. You may see your new baby for the first time in the NICU.

These are some things you can do to make the most of your first moments in the NICU.

- If you are exhausted, take a short nap before going to the NICU.

- Write down questions you want to ask your doctor.

- Eat something if it has been awhile since you had a meal.

- If your partner or support person has already been to the NICU, talk about what you can expect to see and how your baby is doing.

- Use the bathroom before going to the NICU. Women who have just given birth need to urinate frequently and the parent restroom may be outside of the NICU.

- If you have just given birth, go to the NICU by wheelchair. You may feel energized after delivery, but a long walk to the NICU will drain your energy and cut your visit short. The wheelchair is a good way to save energy and it's handy if you feel light-headed and need to sit down.

Your Baby's Care Team

Every NICU has its own team structure and mixture of team players. Each group of professionals is equally important and all work together to care for your baby. You may meet some of these people before, during, or after admission to the NICU.

Nursing Team

Although many people think a nurse is a nurse, nothing could be further from the truth. All nurses have knowledge that provides the foundation for nursing practice, but most also choose an area of specialty.

Neonatal Nurse

A neonatal nurse, usually a registered nurse (RN), is the person who provides most of the moment-to-moment bedside care for your baby (besides you!). A neonatal nurse specializes in the care of newborns and their families. The nurse caring for your baby may have a master's degree or, sometimes, a doctoral degree.

The RN makes recommendations to the physician, neonatal nurse practitioner (NNP), or physician assistant (PA) based on his or her assessment of your baby's condition. The nurse carries out the medical team's orders and notifies them of any changes in your baby's status. In addition, RNs play a key role in parent education and discharge planning.

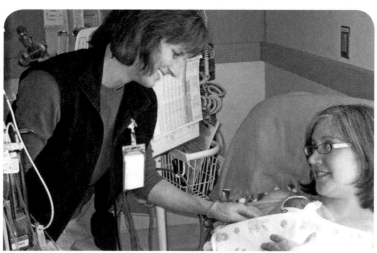

The health care professionals in the neonatal intensive care unit use every opportunity to teach you about your baby's care. This nurse answers a mother's questions and encourages her to talk to her baby.

Courtesy of Seattle Children's Hospital.

> ❝ Thirty-seven days of ups and downs but a lifetime ahead of being grateful for the knowledge of the people around us. ❞
>
> Marnie, mother of **Kellan**

Nursing Education and Leadership

The nursing team is supported by a charge nurse who oversees the nursing operations for each nursing shift. Behind the scenes, you will find a NICU nurse manager who provides supervision and leadership for all of the nursing staff. Many NICUs have a clinical nurse specialist or a nurse educator who serves as a clinical expert, leads staff education, and may lead nursing research, quality improvement, and program development.

Medical Team

Your baby may have more medical professionals than you have encountered in your entire lifetime. In every NICU, a member of the medical team is present in the NICU 24 hours a day and a neonatologist is always on call for that unit.

Neonatologist

A neonatologist is a physician who specializes in the diagnosis and treatment of sick newborns. The neonatologist has completed residency training in pediatrics and then additional training in neonatology. In most NICUs, the neonatologist is the lead physician, referred to as the *attending physician,* and directs the medical care of your baby. The attending physician is responsible for supervising the other members of the medical team.

Fellow

A neonatology fellow is a physician who has completed pediatric residency and is training to become a neonatologist. The fellow works with the attending physician to develop the care plan and supervise the other members of the team.

Resident

A resident is a physician who has graduated from medical school and is completing additional training in a medical specialty (for example, pediatrics, obstetrics, family medicine). The resident assesses your newborn daily and plans the medical care with supervision from the attending physician and fellow.

Pediatric Hospitalist

A pediatric hospitalist is a physician who has completed pediatric residency and has focused his or her practice on the care of babies and children in the hospital. Some hospitalists work in the NICU under the supervision of a neonatologist.

Neonatal Nurse Practitioner

A neonatal nurse practitioner (NNP), also called an advanced registered nurse practitioner (ARNP), is not a doctor but is part of the medical team. An NNP is an RN who has completed advanced training in the care and treatment of sick newborns. An NNP has a master's degree in nursing, and some have a doctoral degree. The NNP works in collaboration with the other members of the medical team to examine, diagnose, and develop the treatment plan.

Physician Assistant

A physician assistant is a licensed medical professional who works under the supervision of a physician to examine, diagnose, and develop the treatment plan.

More Doctors in the House

Your baby's medical team may call on other pediatric specialists to assist them in providing care for your baby. These consultants may be present in your hospital or available on an intermittent basis or by telephone.

- **Cardiac surgeon:** specializes in performing surgery on the heart
- **Cardiologist:** specializes in diagnosis and treatment of heart problems
- **Gastroenterologist:** specializes in treatment of stomach and intestinal problems
- **Geneticist:** studies birth defects and their causes
- **Hematologist:** specializes in diagnosis and treatment of blood problems
- **Neurologist:** specializes in diagnosis and treatment of the nervous system
- **Neurosurgeon:** specializes in surgery of the brain and nervous system
- **Pediatric surgeon:** specializes in performing surgery for newborns and children
- **Pulmonologist:** specializes in diagnosis and treatment of lung conditions and breathing problems
- **Urologist:** specializes in diagnosis and treatment of the urinary tract

> 66 Many of the people who took care of Lucy became our friends. These people will laugh with you, cry with you, teach you to parent, empower you, and cheer you on when you walk out those doors on discharge day. They are there for some of the hardest things you'll ever experience, and they're fantastic. 99
>
> Matthew and Kate, parents of **Lucy**

Support Team

It takes a village to raise a child, and there exists a village in the NICU to support the medical team, nursing team, and your baby. Again, each NICU may have some or all of these team members, and not every baby will require the services of these team members.

- **Case manager/discharge planner:** Follows your baby's hospital course, assists with insurance issues, and helps to organize details for your baby's discharge.
- **Chaplain:** Provides spiritual comfort or guidance, if requested.
- **Financial counselor:** Answers questions about your hospital bills, helps you submit your bill to the appropriate agencies for payment, and sets up a payment plan, if needed.
- **Lactation specialist:** Supports and educates NICU staff, parents, and babies who face breast-feeding challenges.
- **Nutritionist:** Analyzes your baby's energy and nutritional needs and makes suggestions about protein, minerals, and additives for breast milk or formula.
- **Parent-to-parent provider:** Former NICU parent trained to provide support and a listening ear to parents who have little or no experience in the NICU.
- **Pharmacist:** Usually has specific training in neonatal drugs and doses and helps ensure the safety of medications and intravenous nutrition.
- **Respiratory care practitioner:** Specializes in treating problems of the respiratory system. Works under the direction of medical professionals to evaluate and monitor lung function and manage equipment and devices for breathing treatments.

- **Simulation center staff member:** Coordinates education sessions for parents of babies who need special care to help them practice their care skills by using a manikin. This allows learning (and making mistakes) in a safe place and not on a real baby.

- **Social worker:** Helps families cope with stress, deal with financial concerns, use hospital and community resources, and prepare for discharge to home.

- **Students in health care profession programs:** Includes students of nursing, medicine, respiratory therapy, and others. Students do not perform complex procedures and are highly supervised while learning in the NICU.

- **Therapists:** Occupational, physical, speech, massage, and music therapists all have special skills to help your baby's neurologic and physical development.

- **Unit coordinator:** Manages the flow of people, paper, and information into and out of the NICU. Also called a unit secretary, patient services coordinator, or unit clerk.

- **Still more people:** Other personnel include laboratory technicians (trained to obtain blood samples), x-ray technicians, ultrasound technicians, team members who help keep bedside supplies stocked, and housekeepers. Sometimes, staff members are cross-trained, which means they can work in more than one hospital unit and help nurses by taking routine vital signs and transporting patients to different areas of the hospital.

Have We Met Before?

It is possible that in a large children's hospital or regional medical center, you may meet a new physician every week! No wonder you're confused about who is caring for your baby. Until you become familiar with the system, introduce yourself every time you see an unfamiliar face, and never feel shy about asking a team member to identify his or her role on the team. It is your right to know who is caring for your baby. Some NICUs may have a board or an area where the team's pictures and descriptions are posted to help you as well.

Rhythms and Schedules

Scheduling in the NICU is designed to achieve around-the-clock medical and nursing care for patients. The members of the nursing and medical teams work a variety of shifts to ensure appropriate health care professionals are available in the NICU 24 hours a day.

NICU Nurses

Some NICUs use a system called *primary nursing* to allow nurses to get to know specific patients and care for them when they are at work. This is one system that allows a small number of nurses to become most familiar with you and your baby's individual needs. In any case, the nurses who care for your baby are knowledgeable about the plan of care and are interested in helping you learn about your baby and prepare for discharge.

NICU Medical Staff

The members of your baby's medical team may have other responsibilities in the hospital and may change assignments every few weeks. These assignment changes are called *rotations*. This means that every few weeks, you may have a different group of doctors assigned to your baby's care. Neonatal intensive care units use multiple systems to ensure uninterrupted quality care for your baby through these shift changes and rotations.

To find a balance between continuity of care and ensuring your baby's medical team is appropriately rested, most hospital systems have implemented *duty-hour restrictions* for medical professionals. This means the medical team often shares overnight and weekend *on-call* responsibilities so nobody works an excessive number of hours. Hospitals use a variety of different plans to divide work among medical professionals. If you have questions during the night or weekend, you may meet with the medical professionals who are on call for your baby's team. During your stay in the NICU, you will gradually become familiar with all of the members of the medical team.

The Information Playbook

The trust between you and your baby's team is built on communication. Open, direct, and honest communication is vital for families with a baby in the NICU.

Patient Rounds

Many people with different talents are dedicated to caring for your baby. How do all these people coordinate their ideas and plans? The most common and time-honored tradition of team communication is called *patient rounds.* This is when doctors, NNPs, PAs, hospitalists, nurses, respiratory care practitioners, nutritionists, and others involved in your baby's care get together and review the previous day's events and make a plan for the next few days. The purpose of patient rounds is to make certain information is shared accurately, the plan of care moves forward in a coordinated way, and everyone is working toward the day when your baby can go home.

Most NICUs welcome parents to rounds. You are important members of your baby's care team. Your observations of your baby are important to the team's understanding of how your baby is doing. When you share your observations and ideas with the care team during rounds and participate in making decisions, you help the team provide the best care possible for your baby.

> " Participating in rounds was the biggest thing for me. I wrote down my questions as they occurred to me. I also took videos of things I saw so that I could show them what I meant even if the baby didn't happen to be doing it right then. I appreciated it when the attending doc would come in throughout the day and sit down to talk about how things were going. Talking to him one-on-one was far less intimidating than speaking up in rounds. At the same time, the plan was really set during rounds, so it was very important to be there. "
>
> Alex, father of **Pascal**

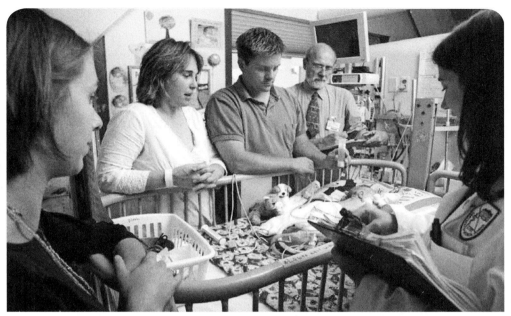

These parents are participating in rounds. Sharing your observations about your baby is very important to providing the best possible care.

Courtesy of George A. Little, MD, FAAP.

The Care Plan

By understanding your baby's care plan, you may better understand daily routines and be able to recognize milestones in your baby's NICU experience.

The care plan guides how and when things are done. The care plan often describes things like what kind of breathing support your baby will receive, how additional oxygen and breathing support will be adjusted, when and how to begin or increase feedings, and when your baby is ready to graduate from an incubator to a crib, and is customized to meet your baby's own medical needs.

It is also important to realize that care plans change. Care plans must be flexible; they depend on your baby's response to treatments and overall condition. Ask often for an update on the care plan. If the plan has changed, you may want to ask, "What is different now that caused this change in the plan?" If your baby's condition has changed but the care plan has not, you may ask, "Why hasn't the plan changed even though my baby hasn't [or has] gotten better?" Asking these simple questions allows you to stay informed, prepare for changes, and participate in your baby's care.

Your baby's medical problems are probably new to you; however, your baby's problems may be common in the NICU. Many NICUs have developed care maps, clinical pathways, or discharge readiness milestones that show the usual path of a common diagnosis. For example, the clinical pathway for a healthy 34 weeks' gestation preterm baby shows what to expect at first and what milestones the baby has to achieve before going home. Seeing what needs to happen in a list or road map may help you understand the road you and your baby are traveling and the path toward coming home.

> 66 All that we read and heard was that you have to be your child's advocate. You need to listen to your gut and share what's on your mind with your child's team. 99
>
> Lisa, mother of **Frankie**

Learning Common Terms, Phrases, and Problems

Learning the words and concepts you hear about in rounds and in the NICU will help you feel more relaxed and comfortable. For efficiency, members of your baby's care team may talk to each other using medical abbreviations and terminology, and sometimes they may forget to translate these terms for you. You are not expected to be a medical expert and should never feel like you have to do homework to know about your baby's care. Do not hesitate to ask your doctor or nurse for explanations. Most NICU providers really enjoy talking with parents and explaining the treatment plan.

Some parents feel more comfortable learning more about NICU terms, phrases, and problems at their own pace. Reading this book will help. Your NICU may also have a parent support program to help you learn about the NICU experience. Talking with other parents who have shared this experience may help. Some NICUs have a parent resource center with books about babies in the NICU and Internet access for finding information. Be cautious about the information you read on the Internet. Anyone can post information, but not all of it will be accurate or even true. Ask for Web site recommendations from a parent educator, a family resource center specialist, or a member of your baby's NICU team. The more you understand, the better you can support your baby.

> " During our weeks in the NICU, I picked up the terminology. I asked questions and I made sure that I understood what was happening at any given time and what the next 'steps' were. Feeling educated helped me feel in control. "
>
> Marnie, mother of **Kellan**

Making Sure You Get the Information You Want and Need

"What if?" Questions

All too often, parents do not ask the "What if?" questions and then become frustrated because their questions have not been addressed. Asking "What if?" questions can make you better informed about the treatment, procedure, or medication in question.

- "What if this drug doesn't work?"
- "What if we decide against surgery?"
- "What if this treatment doesn't work?"

Keep in mind that, at times, a perfect answer doesn't exist. While the knowledge and expertise to care for babies keeps improving, there are times when a decision must be made by carefully weighing the risks and benefits and then choosing what simply feels like the best answer at that time.

What Kind of Information Do You Want?

When you ask your baby's doctor or nurse, "How is my baby today?" you may think it's a simple question, but NICU staff may have difficulty knowing how much and what kind of information you expect. Some parents want specific clinical information, such as laboratory results and ventilator settings. Other parents prefer more general information, such as how well their baby slept or whether their baby is tolerating feedings.

Tell your baby's care providers about the type of information you want and when you want to know it. Give them an example. Do you want to be called immediately with test results, or can you be told when you visit? Do you want to know only the unusual test results, or do you want to know every test result? Be honest with the NICU staff. Don't expect your baby's caregivers to read your mind. Your preferences for information will likely change over time, so remember to update your baby's care team about what you want to know and when.

Scheduling Time With the People You Want to See

As you will learn, there are both many schedules and no schedule in the NICU. The team may usually make rounds at the same time each morning, but then an emergency in the delivery room or with another baby in the NICU changes their schedule. Even if you have been told the neonatologist is usually in the unit at a certain time, do not plan to "catch" the physician for a lengthy chat during patient rounds. A more effective approach is to schedule a time to discuss your baby's progress in person or by telephone. This gives the people involved time to review and organize the most up-to-date information on your baby's care. A scheduled time also decreases the chance you will be interrupted while discussing your questions and concerns.

Care Conferences

Your baby's team may schedule what is called a *care conference* for you, or you may request one. These meetings help familiarize you with team members you may not see daily. Sitting down and talking with several team members (for example, nursing team, medical team, respiratory care practitioners, consultants, social workers) gives you the chance to ask questions of different team members at once, get updates on any big changes in your baby's plan of care, and learn what progress the team is hoping to see from your baby.

When the Unexpected Happens

Sometimes, even the most skilled care team can make a mistake when caring for a baby. When something happens that wasn't expected or planned, it may have been caused by an error. Staying involved in decision-making for your baby is one way to help the team avoid errors—after all, you know your baby better than anyone else. If possible, try to be present during the daily team bedside rounds. This gives you the opportunity to hear what treatments have been planned for your baby as well as to ask questions and provide input. Many parents are not able to devote this amount of time to being in the NICU, but you can still help avoid errors in your baby's care by asking your team to share a daily update of the care plan after rounds.

If you are at your baby's bedside and see something that doesn't seem right, tell your baby's nurse or anyone else on the care team right away at any time of the day or night. If something unexpected has happened, your baby's care team will first want to make sure your baby is safe and any problems are being properly managed. Once your baby's safety is ensured, you will want to learn more about what happened, why, and what will be done to prevent a similar error from occurring again.

Give Yourself Some Time

The NICU is a village, each with its own customs, language, codes of behavior, and "native" habits. You must become part of this new community when your whole world has been turned upside down. You will need some time to adjust to this new environment.

Following your first NICU visits, you may feel overwhelmed and out of place. In time, you will get to know the people caring for your baby and know what they do. With patience, you will develop valuable relationships with them. These are the first important steps toward active involvement in your baby's care.

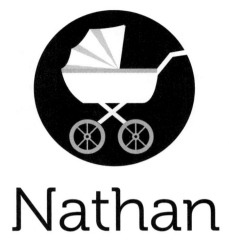

Nathan

Born at 24 weeks 4 days

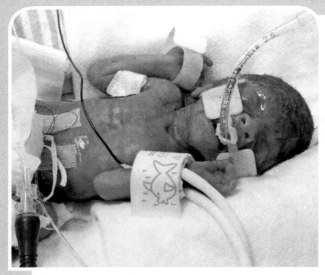

Nathan on his birth day.

At 24 weeks 4 days' gestation, Nathan was born weighing just 1 pound 2 ounces. His premature birth was caused by ruptured membranes 15 weeks into the pregnancy. Miraculously, the pregnancy continued to viability, but due to his early birth, he was born with very immature lungs and the prognosis for long-term survival was grim.

Nathan had much to overcome. On his first day, he suffered from respiratory distress and a collapsed lung. At 1 week, Nathan suffered a bowel perforation, which ultimately resulted in him having surgery at 5 weeks old and just shy of 2 pounds. Almost as soon as he healed from the surgery, Nathan developed a severe form of retinopathy of prematurity (ROP) and was given a 50% chance of going blind. Fortunately, he was able to receive treatment that successfully protected his vision and he can now see just as well as most other kids his age. Almost all of Nathan's major organ systems were affected by his prematurity. Nathan was lucky to have received excellent care during his NICU stay and I will be forever grateful to the wonderful doctors and nurses who cared for him when I couldn't.

Watching my son fight for his life in the hospital every day was incredibly hard, but the many magical moments I experienced with him as he got healthier and stronger kept me going. I will never forget the first time I held him in kangaroo care while he was still on a ventilator, the first time he took a full feed from a bottle with the breast milk I had pumped, and the first time I gave him a bath in a little bucket.

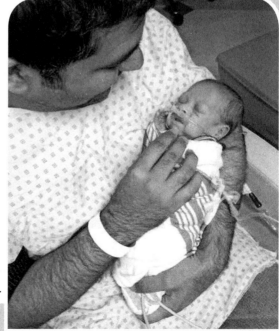

Nathan and his father have a talk.

After 140 days in the NICU, Nathan finally came home. It was a day of overwhelming happiness and gratitude but also one of fear that I was leaving behind the safety net of the NICU and would not know how to properly care for such a tiny being. Thankfully, the transition home went smoothly and I quickly learned how to manage the oxygen tank and apnea monitor that Nathan came home with and stayed on for a few months after leaving the NICU.

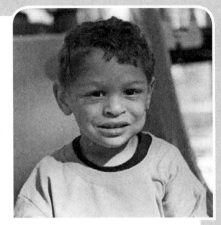

Nathan, at age 3.

Now Nathan is 3 years old, developmentally on schedule in most areas, and an absolute joy in our family's life. Once given less than a 10% chance of survival, Nathan has not only survived, but he's thriving. When he was only 2½ years old, Nathan began reading 3- and 4-letter words, and he's now learning to write some words, too. Nathan is loving, playful, and endlessly curious and has an infectious smile that can light up an entire room.

From the beginning, Nathan showed me his strength and resilience, which continues to inspire me every day. Having been blessed with the miracle of Nathan, my husband and I have established a nonprofit organization to provide support and resources to other families facing the challenges of preterm birth. Despite the harrowing ordeal we went through, we ended up with the greatest outcome we could have ever imagined—a handsome, sweet, and healthy little boy and the opportunity to help others in a meaningful way.

Cheryl and Sunil, parents of Nathan

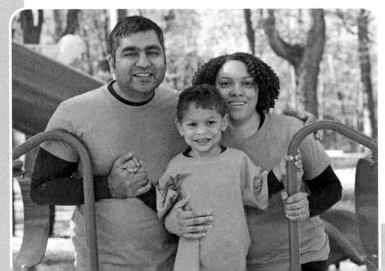

Nathan and his parents.

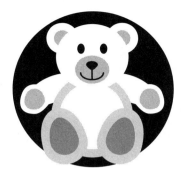

Pascal

Born at 41 weeks 2 days

Pascal was born by C-section and had Apgar scores of 8 and 9. In the recovery room, he was swaddled up in my arms when he turned blue-gray. They checked his oxygen, which seemed OK then. I remember in that moment feeling suspicious of him. I felt disconnected, looking at him from a distance. What was wrong with him? I thought we just had to get to being born, and then he would be OK.

When we moved to the postpartum room, he did it again. That time, his oxygen saturation was in the 60s. They took him to the nursery and then to the NICU. I could see him breathing really, really, really fast. I got to hold him skin-to-skin, with his nasal cannula and IV and monitor cables. When I had to go back to postpartum, I left him my T-shirt so he could still smell me. It felt incredibly wrong to be away from him. His labs strongly suggested infection, so his course of antibiotics was lengthened to 7 days. But that didn't mean we could go home after 7 days.

After a week, he had finished his course of antibiotics and weaned off his high-flow nasal cannula, and we started to work through the discharge process. I watched videos about CPR and safe sleep and set up his first pediatrician appointment. Pascal got set up for his car seat test. Even though he wasn't a preemie, because he'd had breathing problems,

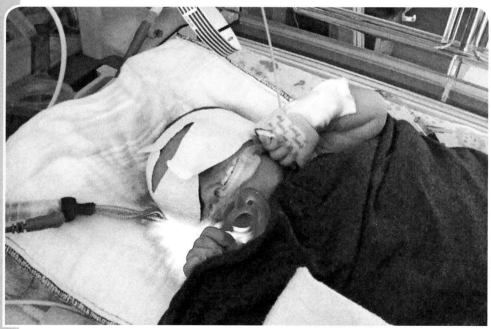

Pascal snuggles with his dad's T-shirt in the NICU during phototherapy treatment.

he had to sit in the seat for 90 minutes without having oxygen desaturations. He failed miserably. Then he failed again. Then again. We ended up staying another 5 days while he got treatment for ongoing breathing problems. It was so hard to be so close to discharge and not be able to go home. You know those stages of grief? I kept going back and forth between acceptance and bargaining. "We don't live very far! I'll get a different stroller! I won't put him in a bouncy seat!" Each time he failed, his team would patiently explain that he wasn't safe to go home yet and that he just needed more time. Finally, on his fourth try, he kept his oxygen levels up, and that afternoon, after 11 days in the NICU, we went home!

Now Pascal is a year old and is pretty healthy, though he gets lots of colds at day care. Even though he's healthy, I still worry a lot when he gets sick, I think because it was so hard for him at the beginning. Our pediatrician understands where I'm coming from and helps me sort through my worry and reassures me about Pascal's health. He loves to climb, bang on boxes, and snuggle on my lap. It's hard to believe just a year ago he needed so much help. I'm so grateful to the team who took care of him and can't wait to take him back to visit so they can see how much he's grown!

Alex, father of Pascal

CHAPTER 3

NICU Equipment and Tests

"Ironically, I had planned for an intervention-free birth before Auggie's early arrival. Because of his early arrival, I am forever grateful for the medical technology and clinical expertise we were afforded and for all of the care he received in the NICU from such dedicated and compassionate nurses and other staff."

*Robyn, mother of **Auggie***

The equipment used for your baby's care in the neonatal intensive care unit (NICU) can be overwhelming for parents. Understanding the basics of NICU technology prepares you to ask questions about your baby's treatment and participate in care. The technology used in the NICU is important for your baby's survival, but it cannot replace the importance of your voice, your touch, and your involvement in your baby's plan of care.

Typical NICU Equipment

Just as the delivery area is set up with basic equipment for birth, the neonatal intensive care unit (NICU) is equipped with technology used to stabilize a sick baby. Each baby's condition determines the type of support needed, but the following equipment and tests are commonly used in the NICU:

Radiant Warmer and Incubator

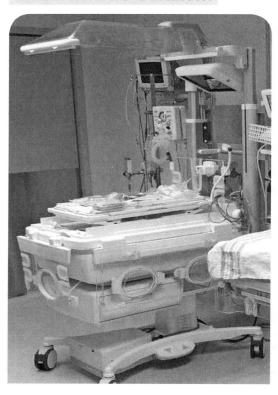

Radiant warmer.

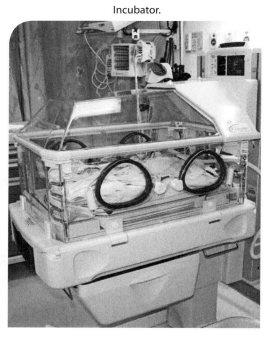

Incubator.

The radiant warmer (left) and incubator (right) are designed to maintain the baby's temperature and enable the NICU team to easily observe and reach the baby. The radiant warmer has overhead heat and allows easy access to the baby from 3 sides. An incubator may have portholes to open or the cover may lift off so you can touch your baby. An incubator maintains a constant warm temperature and humidified air. Most incubators and radiant warmers can also allow thermostat control by measuring the baby's skin temperature through a small sensor taped to your baby's body. This temperature sensor is usually covered by a reflective adhesive material, often a circle of foil or a shiny gold heart. When your baby's skin has warmed to the preset temperature, the heat turns down; when your baby's skin temperature cools, the heat turns back up.

> ❝ The first time I saw my daughter, I remember thinking how amazing it was that she looked like a completely healthy baby...she was just so tiny. Seeing the intubation tube and watching her chest rise and fall so rapidly was heart-wrenching to watch. I just wanted to scoop her up and hold her close, but I couldn't. ❞
>
> Kaitlynn, mother of **Sienna**

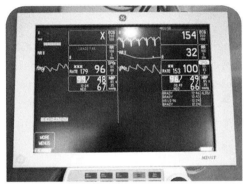

One type of cardiorespiratory monitor.

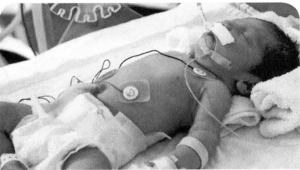

Sienna has 2 round, white electrocardiographic (ECG) leads showing on her chest and tummy; the third ECG lead is near her right shoulder. She is intubated with an endotracheal tube taped to her face and connected to a ventilator. She has an orogastric tube coming from her mouth.

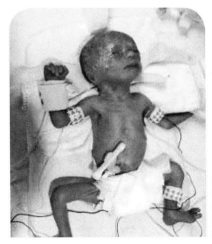

Instead of white ECG leads on her chest, **Frankie** has limb leads visible on her upper arms and leg. The wrapping on her right wrist covers the pulse oximeter sensor to protect it from outside light.

Cardiorespiratory Monitor and ECG (Electrocardiographic) Leads

Most babies in the NICU are placed on a *cardiorespiratory monitor* (sometimes called a *cardiac monitor* or, simply, a *monitor*). This device tracks the baby's vital signs, such as heart rate and breathing rate, and displays these numbers on a screen. This monitor will alert NICU staff to any variation. Three adhesive patches (*ECG leads*) are placed on the baby's chest and abdomen or arms and legs (*limb leads*) and connected by cable to the monitor that displays the information on a screen. The monitor may also display oxygen saturation, if the baby has a pulse oximeter sensor attached, and blood pressure, if the baby has a blood pressure cuff or an umbilical arterial catheter (*UAC*) in use.

Orogastric and Nasogastric Tubes

A thin, flexible tube inserted into your baby's mouth is called an *orogastric (OG)* tube. If it is inserted through the baby's nose, it is called a *nasogastric (NG)* tube. This tube goes down the food pipe (*esophagus*) and into the stomach. The tube may be used to release a buildup of gas and fluids from the baby's stomach (for example, during CPAP), or it may be used to deliver breast milk or formula to a baby who is not yet able to feed from the breast or bottle. When it is used for feeding, it may be called a *feeding tube* or *gavage tube*.

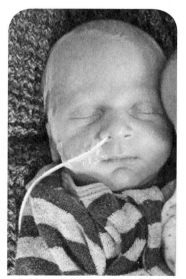

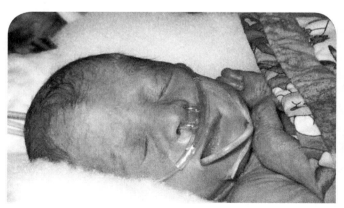

Holland (left) and **Reece** (right) use their orogastric and nasogastric tubes (respectively) for feeding while they mature and learn how to feed from the breast and bottle. When used for feeding, this tube is often called a *feeding tube* or *gavage tube*.

> ❝ One night I was changing Pascal's diaper, and he was flailing around, sticking his feet in the poop, grabbing at his IV, sneezing out his feeding tube, and it was one big giant mess. I think I ended up crying, pleading with him to leave the feeding tube alone, trying to slide it back in before it came out completely or got covered in poop. I could have called for a nurse. Maybe I should have done that, but I wanted so badly to be taking care of him. ❞
>
> Alex, father of **Pascal**

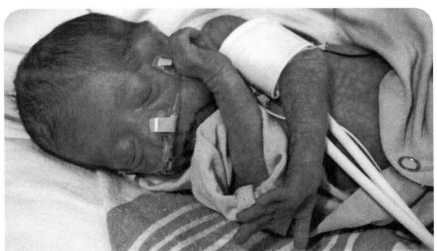

A soft blood pressure cuff wraps around your baby's arm or leg.

Blood Pressure Cuff

Your baby's blood pressure may be taken in much the same way as your own. A small blood pressure cuff is wrapped around your baby's arm or leg, inflates, and measures the blood pressure. If your baby has a UAC, the blood pressure will be displayed on the cardiac monitor. (See Umbilical Arterial Catheter [UAC] for information about the UAC.)

Cerebral Function Monitor

A cerebral function monitor allows the medical team to continuously monitor the brain's electrical activity (brain waves) using small wires attached to the skin on a baby's scalp. The activity is displayed on a screen.

Devices That Support Breathing and Oxygen Status

Many NICU babies require assistance with breathing. The devices described here deliver different kinds of support depending on how much assistance the baby requires. Because of prematurity or illness, your newborn may need to breathe air with a higher concentration of oxygen than is available in "room air," which contains about 21% oxygen. Supplemental oxygen is any amount greater than 21% up to 100%. Supplemental oxygen, unless it is being used for a short period or set at a very low flow, is warmed and humidified. It can be given in several different ways.

Ventilator and Endotracheal Tube

A respirator (also called a ventilator) assists breathing for a baby who is having trouble breathing on her own. There are many different types of ventilators, and each one works a little differently. The assisted breath is delivered through an *endotracheal (ET) tube* inserted into the baby's windpipe (*trachea*). A ventilator can be adjusted to give the correct air–oxygen mixture, the correct size of the breath (pressure and duration), and the correct number of breaths per minute, depending on the baby's needs.

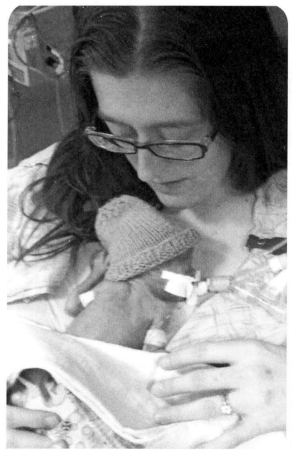

Robyn holds **Auggie** for the first time when he's about 2 weeks old. He is intubated, and the long tubing over Robyn's shoulder connects the endotracheal tube that is secured to his face to the ventilator nearby. The limb leads that connect to the cardiac monitor are clearly visible around his upper arms.

Nasal Cannula

A *nasal cannula* is tubing that wraps around your baby's head and has prongs that fit into the baby's nose. A cannula can be used to deliver air or oxygen in a variety of ways.

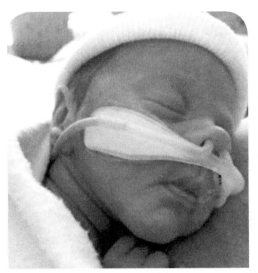
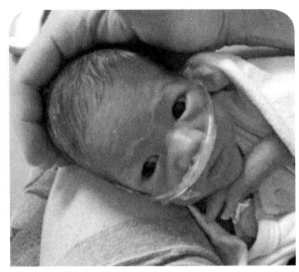

A cannula is the device used to deliver air, oxygen, CPAP, or noninvasive ventilation. On the left, **Lucy** wears one style of nasal cannula. The prongs are clearly visible in her nose. On the right, **Henry** wears a different style nasal cannula.

" Take lots of pictures and videos and sneak a few of those tiny diapers to show people. They are blown away when they see the size of those diapers. "

Lisa, mother of **Frankie**

Continuous Positive Airway Pressure (CPAP)

A baby with CPAP breathes on her own, but CPAP keeps a steady stream of low air pressure in her airway. This helps keep the tiny air sacs in her lungs from collapsing after each breath, making it easier for her to breathe. (See Chapter 5 for more information.) Most babies on CPAP also have an *orogastric (OG) tube* inserted through the mouth into the stomach. It is used to release the air that might get into the stomach and interfere with breathing.

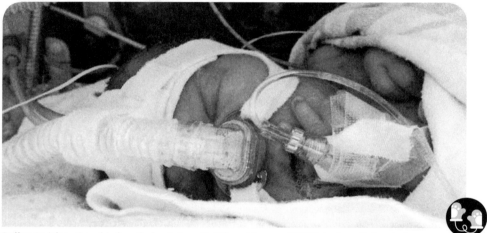

Bailey Jo (above) and **Lukas** (below) show 2 different types of CPAP devices. Bailey Jo has an intravenous line in her hand that she holds near her mouth. Lukas has an orogastric tube in his mouth.

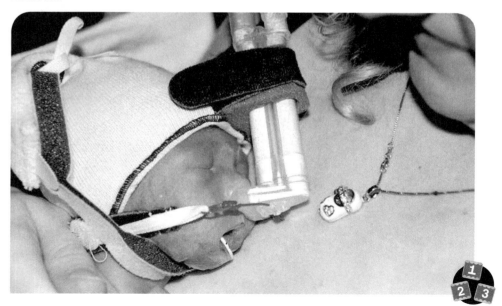

Pulse Oximeter

Pulse oximetry may have been used in the delivery room if your baby needed resuscitation or supplemental oxygen. In the NICU, the pulse oximeter sensor wraps around your baby's hand, wrist, or foot. It uses a red light to measure the amount of oxygen attached to the hemoglobin molecules in your baby's blood. The measurement, called *oxygen saturation,* is displayed on the pulse oximeter screen along with your baby's heart rate. If your baby's oxygen saturation is outside the target range, your baby's nurse or respiratory care practitioner may make an adjustment to her respiratory equipment.

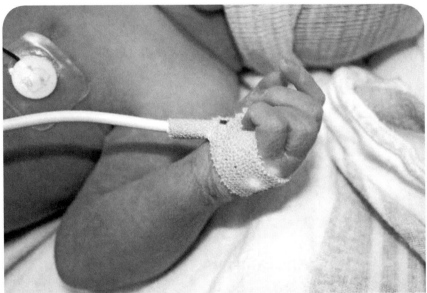

The pulse oximeter shines a painless red light onto the baby's skin. The sensor is often covered with a soft cloth wrap to keep bright light in the room from interfering with the pulse oximeter signal.

> ❝ I remember the sounds of the NICU especially. The monitors were fussy and would lose his oxygen saturation. I got the hang of interpreting whether it was a real problem or just the monitor looking for a signal. ❞
>
> Alex, father of **Pascal**

Carbon Dioxide Transcutaneous Monitor

A *transcutaneous monitor* (*TCM*) is used for monitoring carbon dioxide levels in the bloodstream. The TCM sensor lies on your baby's skin and warms the area under the sensor to "read" the amount of carbon dioxide in the blood. This can help determine if the baby needs additional help with breathing. Because of the warmth of the sensor, the TCM may leave a temporary red circle on your baby's skin.

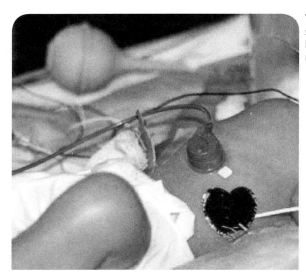

The transcutaneous monitor uses a round, plastic sensor that lies on the baby's skin. The shiny heart holds the temperature sensor in place for the radiant warmer or incubator.

Lines and Catheters

Because most babies in the NICU require fluids, medications, and nutrition via a blood vessel for some time after birth, they require some type of intravenous line or catheter. The type of device used depends on how long and for what purpose it is needed.

Intravenous Line

An *intravenous line* (often simply called an *IV*) is used to give your baby fluids, sugar, protein, salts and minerals (for example, sodium and potassium), and medications. Your baby's IV may be placed in a vein in her hand or lower arm, foot or lower leg, or scalp. The IV can easily move out of place, allowing the IV fluid to leak into the tissue. This is called an *infiltrated IV*. If this happens, it must be taken out (*discontinued*) and restarted at another site. The nurse safeguards the IV so it functions at one site for as long as possible. Even under the best circumstances, an IV may last only a day or two.

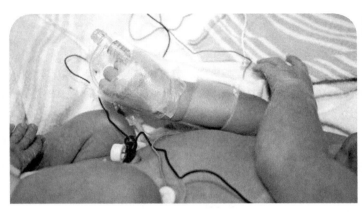

An intravenous line is placed into a vein near the skin surface.

Arterial Line

If the NICU team needs continuous monitoring of your baby's blood pressure, they may place an *arterial line*. An arterial line is a special catheter that is threaded into an artery and then attached to an electronic monitor. In the NICU, arterial lines are frequently placed into an artery in the wrist or ankle.

Umbilical Arterial Catheter (UAC)

A *UAC* is inserted into one of the 2 arteries that are easily visible at the end of the umbilical cord and advanced until it reaches a large artery (the *aorta*). A UAC is placed if your baby requires frequent blood testing or continuous blood pressure measurement.

Umbilical Venous Catheter (UVC)

An *umbilical venous catheter* (*UVC*) is inserted into the umbilical vein, easily visible at the end of the umbilical cord, and advanced until it reaches a larger vein just inside the baby's abdomen. An emer-

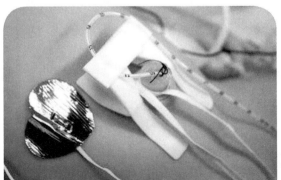

gency UVC may be inserted if your baby needs to have fluids or medications infused during resuscitation. A UVC may also be inserted if your baby needs an IV for more than a few days.

An umbilical catheter is a thin tube that can be threaded into an umbilical artery (umbilical arterial catheter) or an umbilical vein (umbilical venous catheter). This umbilical catheter is often secured with a "bridge" of white tape. The shiny foil heart on the left holds the temperature sensor in place on the skin.

> Holland had a really awesome day today. The line in Holland's belly button was taken out and a PICC line was put in and worked great with just one attempt. I was very happy about that because I just hate when they have to be poked!
>
> Billie, mother of **Holland** and **Eden**

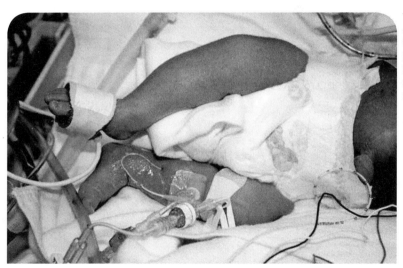

The peripherally inserted central catheter (PICC line) is the thin white tubing on this baby's left leg. This baby also has a pulse oximeter sensor and sensor cover on her right foot.

Peripherally Inserted Central Catheter (PICC line)

A *peripherally inserted central catheter* (*PICC* ["pick"]) *line*, or *central line*, is used when your baby needs an IV for longer than a few days. It is inserted into the arm or leg and threaded into a larger blood vessel deep inside the body. The PICC line is used to give medicines, fluids, and nutrients over a longer period, usually a week or more.

> ❝ One of my regrets was declining the PICC line when it was offered. A PICC line seemed invasive and scary, but that IV was really hard to keep in. How does a newborn have enough coordination to gnaw on his own IV? He was a big chunky baby and IV placements were frequent and difficult. ❞
>
> Alex, father of **Pascal**

Basic NICU Tests

The NICU team uses many different tests to get information about your baby's health.

Imaging Tests

Radiographs

Radiographs (also called x-rays) are an important diagnostic tool in the NICU. Radiographs are used to confirm the correct position of tubes and catheters, such as the endotracheal tube and umbilical catheter, if one is in place. Radiographs also allow care providers to assess the condition of the lungs.

Although your baby is exposed to a certain amount of radiation with every radiograph, the amount is carefully controlled in relation to your baby's size and weight. Unnecessary radiographs are avoided. If the baby's genital area is in the primary x-ray beam, it is shielded with a lead cover.

Ultrasound

Just like ultrasound tests used during pregnancy, an *ultrasound* may be used to look at various organs, including your baby's brain, heart, liver, and kidneys. Sometimes, the ultrasound machine will be used to help guide the medical team as they perform procedures. The ultrasound machine uses sound waves instead of radiation.

Blood Tests

Blood Culture

If the team suspects your baby may have an infection, a sample of blood will be taken and sent for a *blood culture*. The blood sample is placed in a bottle and sent to the laboratory, where it is watched for several days for signs of bacterial (or fungal) growth. Bacteria often take several days to grow (1–3 days), and fungus may take longer (a week or more). If there is no sign of bacterial growth, the culture is called *negative*. In this case, negative is a good thing. Viruses are different from bacteria and require special kinds of culture methods. At times, your team may obtain blood or other samples for viral culture.

Blood Gas

A *blood gas* is a test that uses a small amount of blood to check the levels of oxygen, carbon dioxide, and acid. The blood can be sampled from different sources. Sometimes, it requires health care professionals to use a syringe and needle to get blood from an artery. This is called an *arterial blood gas (ABG)*. Other times, a *venous blood gas* may be obtained with a syringe and a needle from a vein. A cap gas (short for *capillary blood gas* or CBG), which is obtained by pricking your baby's heel with a small puncture device, may be sufficient. If blood gas levels are needed frequently, the team may insert a catheter into a larger blood vessel and obtain the sample through the catheter, avoiding the need to puncture your baby's skin for each sample.

Blood gas results are commonly used to help the team check your baby's lung function and make adjustments to the ventilator. A blood gas test can also give the team valuable information about your baby's metabolism, hydration, and nutrition.

Complete Blood Cell Count

A *complete blood cell count* (CBC) is a test to measure the different components of your baby's blood, including the amount of red blood cells (*hematocrit* and *hemoglobin*), white blood cells, and platelets. Red blood cells carry oxygen to tissues. When they are low, it means the baby has *anemia*. White blood cells are used to fight infection. If they are very low or very high, it may be a sign of infection. Platelets are used to make blood clot and control bleeding.

Electrolytes

Electrolytes (sometimes called *lytes*) measure the balance of salts and minerals in your baby's blood. Measuring electrolytes helps the team make adjustments to the fluids and nutrition she receives and assess how well her kidneys are functioning.

Glucose (Blood Sugar)

Blood glucose measures the amount of sugar in your baby's blood. Frequently, it is tested at the bedside using a small drop of blood from your baby's heel. If the number is unusually high or low, a sample may be obtained from a blood vessel and sent to the laboratory for more precise analysis.

Newborn Metabolic Screening (State Screening)

All newborns in the United States have a blood sample obtained shortly after birth. The blood is placed onto a special piece of paper. The sample is sent to a central laboratory, usually in the same state, and tested for a wide range of inherited diseases. Many of these tests are looking for rare but important abnormalities of hormones and metabolism. It is common for babies in the NICU to have temporary abnormalities on these tests called *false positives*. If a component of the metabolic screen is abnormal, someone from the laboratory may contact you and your baby's doctor by phone. Your doctor will explain the test result and describe the plan for follow-up.

Sepsis Evaluation

Right after birth, or later if your baby's condition changes, the care team may need to decide if your baby has an infection. Looking for laboratory signs of infection is often called a *sepsis evaluation*. The team will obtain a variety of blood tests (as described previously) and, possibly, urine and spinal fluid samples.

Spinal Fluid

If the team suspects your baby may have an infection, they may also want to obtain a sample of *cerebral spinal fluid*. If the spinal fluid is infected, it is called *meningitis*. The sample is obtained by inserting a very small needle into the baby's back between her vertebrae. This procedure is called a *lumbar puncture*.

Urine Tests

Kidneys are very sensitive to changes in the body. The amount of your baby's urine and what is in it can tell the NICU team much about your baby's general condition and progress after birth. If a urine sample is needed, a specially designed plastic bag may be taped over your baby's labia or penis and scrotum. When the baby urinates, the urine collects in the bag and is sent to the laboratory for analysis. This type of urine collection is called a *clean catch* and is used to check the urine for sugar, salts, or blood.

If infection is a concern, a urine culture may be done. The urine sample may be collected by inserting a small sterile catheter into the baby's bladder through the opening where urine comes out (the baby's *urethra*) and withdrawing the urine. Sometimes, it can be very difficult to insert a sterile catheter into a small baby's urethra. In this case, another method is used that involves inserting a needle through the baby's lower abdomen and directly into the bladder. This technique is called a *suprapubic* or *bladder tap*.

The Importance of Parenting

The NICU you enter today is very different from the NICU of even a few years ago. Advances in respiratory care, monitoring, and diagnostic techniques have been incredible. This technology can be overwhelming for parents, but the NICU team will answer your questions, help you get acquainted with your baby despite the wires and cables, and guide you as you learn about equipment and procedures in the NICU. Soon, you'll know the purpose of each device and what each sound means. Paying attention to your baby is more important than watching the monitors!

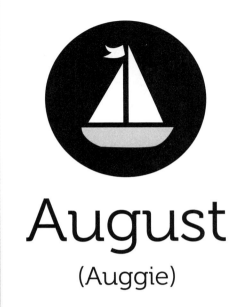

August

(Auggie)

Born at 24 weeks

Auggie was born in 2013 at 24 weeks of gestation. He weighed 1 pound 13 ounces at birth and spent his first 131 days of life in the Infant Special Care Unit.

Just before the 24-week mark, I started experiencing some very faint discharge. At first I thought I was overreacting and that it was likely a normal reaction of my body to a pregnancy at that stage. Thankfully, I listened to that little voice in the back of my head and called my midwife. It was in that moment that everything related to our birth plan unraveled, every vision or plan for a healthy, uncomplicated birth experience vanished. I was admitted to the hospital and soon after, I had a placental abruption and an emergency C-section.

Auggie was handed off to the neonatology team for resuscitation and they worked quickly to save him. I don't think we fully understood until much later just how important those first few minutes were in determining whether he would survive.

We would not hold our son for 2 weeks and spent the next 4½ months making daily visits to the NICU to see him, multiple calls per day to get updates on his progress, and taking it all one day at a time. It was the longest 131 days of our life.

The way we became parents to Auggie was hard; it was emotionally exhausting, and that lasted well after the physical pain from the aftermath of his birth. It's hard on marriages to start your life-changing journey as parents while your baby is still in the NICU. I had a lot of guilt and lingering emotional stress and didn't quite know how to process it all.

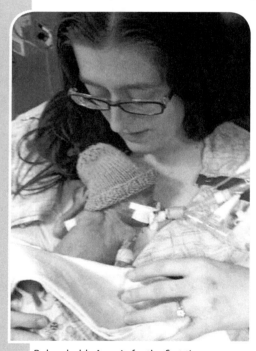

Robyn holds Auggie for the first time.

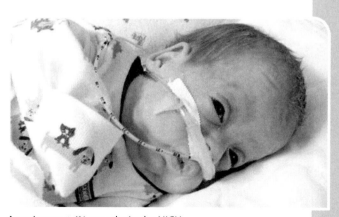

Auggie spent 4½ months in the NICU.

My husband processed his emotions differently, so it was a strain and it was frustrating to both of us to understand one another's vastly different expressions. I felt guilty, as though it were somehow my fault that my baby was born in such a fragile state, with his life in the balance. I was hard on myself.

One thing I wish I knew earlier on during our journey was to ask for help and to accept that post-traumatic stress disorder (PTSD) is very much something that NICU parents can experience. There were horrible flashbacks and guttural cries, initially, thinking about the horrible nightmare of his birth and the short time leading up to his birth. We didn't know if he would live or if his quality of life would be "good" if he did live. I still find it difficult to relate to women who have uncomplicated, full-term births. I didn't experience a third trimester of pregnancy.

Another thing I have forgiven myself for, but didn't at the time, was my inability to love my son in the first few weeks. At 24 weeks' gestation, he didn't look like the babies you see in pictures or on social media. It was a defense mechanism, I think. I didn't have anyone in my social network who had had a baby so early, or even preterm at all. That was isolating.

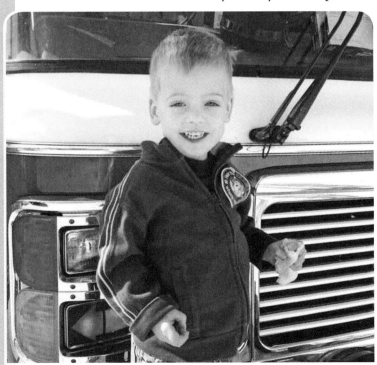

There was so much anticipation and buildup for our son's discharge from the NICU that by the time the day arrived, I was surprised by my sudden sadness to leave the place I so desperately wanted to flee. I was sad to leave the nurses, who we could never thank enough for their care of our child. Bringing Auggie home had its own challenges, however; we worried constantly those first few months about his development, whether he was getting the right nutrition, and whether he'd contract some illness.

Auggie, at age 2½ years.

Three years later, I still marvel at his auspicious beginnings in life and how remarkably he's overcome all of the hurdles in his way. We will admit that we have one of the best-case outcomes; Auggie does not have any lingering physical or mental developmental delays. I'm always cognizant of the fact that there are many NICU families dealing with more severe complications of their children's early births. That's never lost on me. I'd do it all over again because I have this amazing, smart, funny, curious, friendly, compassionate little person who is our son. I'm in awe of him, that we get to be his. He's like the best gift that I never quite feel I deserve.

Robyn, mother of Auggie

CHAPTER 4

Common Medical Problems

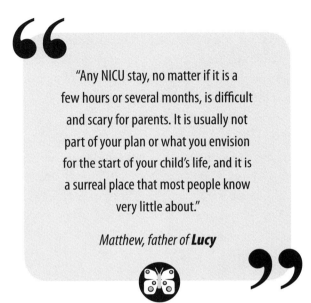

"Any NICU stay, no matter if it is a
few hours or several months, is difficult
and scary for parents. It is usually not
part of your plan or what you envision
for the start of your child's life, and it is
a surreal place that most people know
very little about."

Matthew, father of **Lucy**

This chapter will help explain some of the medical problems that babies will have in the neonatal intensive care unit (NICU). Preterm and full-term newborns can have these problems. Some of the problems that are specific to preterm babies are discussed in the next chapter.

Some babies will never have any of the problems discussed in this chapter, while others may face many challenges. The descriptions in this chapter are brief and include some of the most common findings and treatments for each problem. Each baby is different, and your baby's situation may differ a little or a lot from the descriptions you read here. Your NICU team can provide you with more specific details about your baby.

Problems With Breathing

Transient Tachypnea of the Newborn (TTN)

During development, the fetal lungs are filled with fluid, not air. During the process of labor and birth, most of this fluid is removed. *Transient tachypnea of the newborn* (*TTN*), or "wet lung," develops when fluid remains in the newborn's lungs after birth. Babies born by cesarean or rapid vaginal delivery are at increased risk for developing TTN.

Potential Problems Caused by TTN

Fluid in the lungs makes it hard for your baby to breathe and may cause fast breathing (*tachypnea*), labored breathing (resulting in *retractions of the chest wall*), and moaning or grunting sounds with breathing. The additional work of breathing is tiring and makes it hard to get enough oxygen and get rid of carbon dioxide. Rapid breathing also makes sucking and swallowing difficult and may make it very hard for your baby to eat.

Diagnosis and Treatment of TTN

A chest x-ray (*radiograph*) may look hazy and show signs of fluid in the lungs. Some babies with TTN require additional oxygen or a small amount of continuous pressure given through a mask or small prongs in the baby's nose (continuous positive airway pressure, or *CPAP*) to help with breathing. Transient tachypnea of the newborn and pneumonia can appear very similar on a chest radiograph, so your baby may receive antibiotics if the medical team considers pneumonia a possibility. Your baby may need intravenous (*IV*) fluids until his breathing slows down. Usually, TTN resolves within a couple of days and does not lead to any lasting problems.

Meconium Aspiration Syndrome (MAS)

Meconium is a sterile, dark-green, sticky substance produced in the fetal bowel and passed in the baby's first few stools (bowel movements) after birth. Sometimes, the baby passes meconium while still in the uterus. In other words, the baby poops for the first time in the uterus before he is born. The poop makes the amniotic fluid, which is usually clear, a greenish-brown color. This is called *meconium-stained amniotic fluid* (*MSAF*).

Meconium-stained amniotic fluid is more common when the pregnancy goes late (*post-term*) and may be a sign of fetal distress. After the fetus passes meconium, the fetus may get MSAF into his mouth and airway before or right after birth. Babies who get a large amount of meconium into their lungs can have severe breathing problems after birth. This condition is called *meconium aspiration syndrome* (*MAS*). About 10% of all babies pass meconium in the amniotic fluid, but only a small number of these babies have breathing problems.

Resuscitation of Babies With Meconium-Stained Amniotic Fluid

Until recently, if a baby with MSAF was born limp and not breathing, a tube was inserted into his windpipe (*endotracheal intubation*) and suction was applied to remove meconium. Research has not shown that *intubation* and *tracheal suction* prevent MAS, and routinely inserting a tube into the windpipe for suction is no longer recommended.

Symptoms of MAS

After birth, the dark-colored meconium may temporarily stain the baby's skin, fingernails, or umbilical cord a greenish color. Babies who have inhaled meconium into their lungs may need help to breathe after birth. They may have rapid breathing (*tachypnea*), blue color of the body and around the mouth (*cyanosis*), widely opened nostrils with each breath (*nasal flaring*), and increased work of breathing resulting in the drawing in of the chest wall with each breath (*retractions*).

Potential Complications of MAS

The complications of meconium aspiration will depend on the baby's degree of distress before birth and the severity of MAS.

Mild meconium aspiration usually resolves with few problems. Babies with mild meconium aspiration may need extra oxygen and IV fluids for several hours to days following birth. If your baby is breathing rapidly, feeding may be delayed and IV fluid may be necessary.

More severe cases of MAS can make a baby very sick. Meconium is irritating to the lungs, and although it is sterile, it may encourage an infection. Some babies may develop a problem called *persistent pulmonary hypertension of the newborn* (*PPHN*), described later in this chapter. Babies with severe MAS may need a breathing tube inserted in their windpipe (*endotracheal intubation*) and a ventilator to assist breathing, antibiotics, and treatments to relax the blood vessels in their lungs. Giving *surfactant* into the lungs may help improve lung function. (See Chapter 5.) Sometimes, babies are given oxygen mixed with a gas called *nitric oxide* to help relax the blood vessels in the lungs (see the Treatment for PPHN section for more information about nitric oxide). Meconium may trap air in the tiny breathing sacs of the lung (*alveoli*), causing them to rupture and leak air into the spaces around the lung. Babies with the most severe MAS may need to be transferred to a higher level, specialized NICU for a temporary form of heart–lung bypass called *extracorporeal membrane oxygenation* (*ECMO*) (explained later in this chapter).

Air Leaks

When a baby has trouble breathing, one possible complication is an *air leak*. This occurs when air ruptures one or more of the breathing sacs of the lung (*alveoli*) and air leaks into the spaces around the lung tissue. Air that collects between the lung and rib cage is called a *pneumothorax* and may cause the lung to collapse.

Babies at Risk for Air Leaks

Some healthy babies will develop an air leak when they inflate their lungs with their very first breaths after birth. Others will develop an air leak because they have excess fluid or meconium in their lungs. Babies who need breathing support from CPAP or a ventilator have a higher risk of developing an air leak because of the mechanical pressure within their lungs. Preterm babies are also at more risk because their lungs are stiffer at birth.

Signs of an Air Leak

Some babies with an air leak have no signs or only mild rapid breathing (*tachypnea*). Other babies show more signs of distress, including low heart rate (*bradycardia*), labored breathing, low blood pressure (*hypotension*), and decreased oxygen saturation.

Diagnosis of Air Leaks

A chest radiograph is used to diagnose air leaks. If a baby suddenly has respiratory distress, a bright light may be shined on his chest to look for a "glow" that indicates a collection of air outside the lung. This procedure is called *transillumination*. Although the result is not as specific as a chest radiograph, transillumination can usually be done more quickly in an emergency than a chest radiograph.

Treatment for Air Leaks

Newborns with a small air leak and no significant breathing problems do not require any treatment. If the air leak causes more significant breathing problems, the air can be removed by inserting a needle into the chest and pulling out the air with a syringe. This procedure is called *needle aspiration* or *needle thoracentesis*. If there is concern the air may keep leaking, a thin plastic or silicone tube (*chest tube*) attached to a suction device can be left in the chest to remove the leaking air. In most cases, the damaged alveoli repair themselves within several days and the chest tube can be removed.

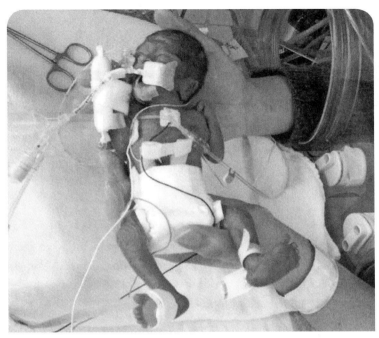

Nathan's mother holds him at first by putting her hands through the incubator portholes. "Nathan had much to overcome. On his first day, he suffered from respiratory distress and a collapsed lung."

*Cheryl, mother of **Nathan***

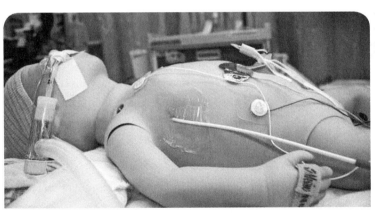

This is a manikin used for NICU training. Note the white tube inserted into the "baby's" chest. This is a chest tube, used to treat a pneumothorax.

Persistent Pulmonary Hypertension of the Newborn (PPHN)

Before birth, the fetus does not use his lungs and the blood vessels leading to the lungs are tightly squeezed (*constricted*). After birth, babies take their first breaths, fill their lungs with air, and the blood vessels normally relax. *Persistent pulmonary hypertension of the newborn* occurs when the blood vessels do not relax and blood cannot get into the lungs. This decreases the oxygen supply to the newborn's body and can be a life-threatening problem.

Babies who have trouble with breathing after birth are at risk of PPHN. The signs of PPHN look a lot like signs of other major illnesses. Your baby may have difficulty breathing, have low blood pressure, or look pale, blue, or blotchy (*mottled*).

Diagnosis of PPHN

If your baby requires very high amounts of additional oxygen to maintain normal blood oxygen levels, PPHN may be suspected. A cardiac ultrasound (*echocardiogram*) is often done to look at how well the heart is working. The echocardiogram looks at how well the blood is flowing to the lungs and measures the pressure in the heart and major blood vessels.

Treatment for PPHN

The goals of treatment are to relax the blood vessels in the lungs and improve oxygen levels in the blood. Babies often need help from a ventilator. There are many different kinds of ventilators. The medical team may use a special ventilator called a *high-frequency ventilator* that provides very rapid breaths with vibrations or small puffs of air. Medications may be needed to help to raise your baby's blood pressure (*vasopressors* or *pressors*) or help him to sleep and relieve any discomfort.

Other possible treatments for severe PPHN include the use of *inhaled nitric oxide* or *ECMO*.

Nitric Oxide

Nitric oxide is an important chemical in the body that helps regulate blood pressure. When breathed into the lungs, nitric oxide relaxes the blood vessels in the lungs and can improve oxygen entry. Note that nitric oxide sounds similar *but is not the same as* nitrous oxide or "laughing gas."

Extracorporeal Membrane Oxygenation

Babies are considered for ECMO (pronounced "EK-mo") if other treatments have not been successful. Extracorporeal membrane oxygenation is a type of temporary heart–lung bypass that allows the baby's lungs (and sometimes the heart) to rest so they can recover. The machine used for ECMO is similar to the machine used for open-heart surgery and requires 1 or 2 large tubes (*cannulas*) to be surgically placed in large blood vessels in the baby's neck. Extracorporeal

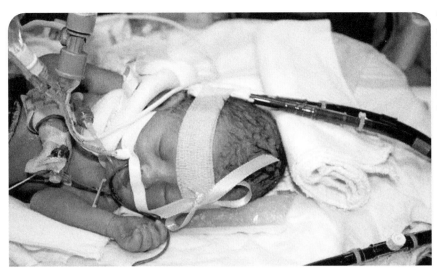

This baby is on extracorporeal membrane oxygenation (ECMO). The large tube that shows above the baby's head is the cannula that is placed in a large vessel of her neck.

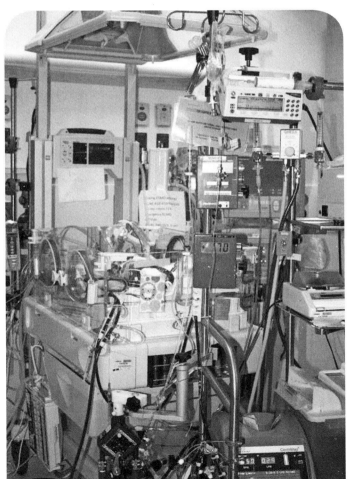

The typical amount of equipment at the bedside of a newborn on ECMO.

membrane oxygenation is surgically and technically complex and is not available at every NICU; therefore, if your baby requires ECMO, he may be transferred to a higher level, specialized NICU.

When a baby is on ECMO, his lungs are no longer the main way that he breathes, but he may still remain intubated and receive some breathing support from a ventilator at low settings. Babies need to remain quiet and may receive pain medications, as well as sedatives, to ensure comfort. How long a newborn remains on ECMO varies depending on his condition and on the recovery of heart and lung function. Most newborns average 5 to 7 days on ECMO, but some will need ECMO for much longer.

Although ECMO can be lifesaving, there are risks associated with being on ECMO. These include bleeding, forming of blood clots, and kidney failure. The blood vessel used for ECMO cannulas may be permanently blocked after ECMO, and this can pose a risk for future problems.

Problems With Infections

Our immune system protects us from infection. The body has many defense mechanisms to prevent things like bacteria and viruses from invading. Because the defense mechanisms of babies are still immature, newborns are at greater risk for developing an infection than are older children or adults.

Why Babies Are at Risk

The skin and mucous membranes that line the respiratory system and gut help to keep potential invaders out. If foreign bodies get past these barriers, white blood cells, antibodies, and other substances in the blood are called into action to find and attack them.

Some risk factors for infection can be identified before the baby is born. If there are signs of infection in the amniotic fluid during labor or the baby is born preterm, the risk of early newborn infection is significantly increased. Preterm newborns have a greater risk of developing infections during their first weeks of life because all of their defense mechanisms are immature. Their skin does not form a complete barrier, their white blood cells are not as effective at killing invaders, and they have fewer antibodies in their blood. Babies receive antibodies from their mother during the third trimester of pregnancy, and many preterm babies are born before these antibodies are transferred across the placenta.

Babies in the NICU, in general, are at risk for infection during their hospital stay. Some of the medical equipment and procedures that babies in the NICU need to survive, including breathing tubes, feeding tubes, and IV lines, interfere with their protective barriers and increase the risk of infection.

Risk Factors for Early Newborn Infection

- Prematurity
- Preterm or prolonged rupture of amniotic membranes
- Maternal fever
- Infection of the placenta and amniotic fluid (*chorioamnionitis*)
- Maternal colonization with group B β-hemolytic streptococcus (*group B strep*)
- Previous baby with infection in the newborn period

Signs of Possible Infection

- Difficulty breathing
- Breathing pauses (*apnea*)
- Limp muscle tone (*hypotonia*)
- Lack of energy (*lethargy*)
- Irritability or fussiness
- Seizures
- Vomiting
- Pale, mottled, or blotchy skin
- Low body temperature
- Fever
- Low blood pressure (*hypotension*)
- Low blood sugar (*hypoglycemia*)
- High blood sugar (*hyperglycemia*)
- Rapidly appearing yellow skin (*jaundice*)

Signs of Infection

Babies who are coming down with an infection often show general signs of illness or signs that mimic other problems. These may be subtle or quite dramatic, depending on the severity and type of infection and the type of organism causing it.

Diagnosis of Infection

If the NICU team suspects your baby has an infection, they will do a *sepsis evaluation*. They take samples of your baby's body fluids and send them to the laboratory to see if bacteria can be identified. Depending on your baby's age and signs of infection, they may take samples of blood, urine, and spinal fluid for culture testing. The laboratory monitors the cultures and will contact the NICU team if there are signs of bacterial growth. It commonly takes 12 to 48 hours in the laboratory before a culture shows any signs of bacterial growth. If nothing grows, the culture is called *negative*. Other blood tests, such as a blood cell count, and radiographs of the chest or belly may also be done. At times, the team may be concerned about less common types of infections, including very slow growing bacteria, viruses, and fungi (yeast). If the team suspects one of these infections, they may send additional samples for cultures and other tests.

> Holland took a turn for the worse when she was about a week old. Her platelet count dropped rather suddenly, and the doctors suspected she had an infection. The next 2 days were really long, stressful days, and we did not get a lot of good news. It was very disheartening. Finally, on day 4, Holland's platelet count improved! Through it all, Holland was a really tough cookie. All of her tiny little parts continued to function and she plugged right along.
>
> Billie, mother of **Holland** and **Eden**

Treatment for Infection

The treatment for bacterial infection is antibiotics—medications that are effective against bacteria. First, your baby receives antibiotics that are effective against many different types of bacteria (*broad-spectrum antibiotics*). As caregivers learn more about the type of bacteria causing your baby's infection, they may give a more specific antibiotic. If your baby needs treatment for a virus or fungus, other medications will be added to the treatment plan.

Supportive care is also provided to increase your baby's ability to fight the infection. A warm environment, IV fluids, medicines to maintain normal blood pressure, adequate nutrition (oral or IV), and oxygen or assisted breathing, as needed, are examples of supportive care.

Two Specific Infections: Group B β-Hemolytic Streptococcus and Central Line–Associated Bloodstream Infection

Group B β-Hemolytic Streptococcus

Group B β-*hemolytic streptococcus* (*GBS;* also called *group B strep*) is a type of bacteria found in the birth canal or rectum in about 10% to 30% of healthy women. This organism does not usually cause any symptoms or illness in the mother but, in some cases, may be responsible for maternal urinary tract infection or infection of the amniotic membranes that surround the baby before birth (*chorioamnionitis*).

Pregnant women are screened for GBS at about 35 to 37 weeks of pregnancy. If a pregnant woman carries this organism in her vagina or rectum, she will receive antibiotics during labor to help prevent the spread of GBS to her baby. Without antibiotics, some babies born after labor starts to mothers with GBS bacteria will develop a serious infection. This overall risk is about 1 in 100 babies, but the risk to an individual baby is much lower or much higher than that, depending on how long before birth the mother's water is broken and whether or not the mother develops a fever during labor. The risk is even higher if the baby is born preterm, if the mother has a large amount of GBS bacteria present, if she had urinary tract infections with GBS, or if she has had a previous baby with GBS infection. With antibiotics in labor, the risk of the baby becoming infected is decreased almost 100-fold. If a mother undergoes a planned cesarean delivery before labor starts and before her water breaks, the risk of GBS infection is very low and antibiotics are not given.

Group B strep infection in the newborn can cause blood infection, pneumonia, a severe whole body reaction to infection (*sepsis*), or infection of the spinal fluid (*meningitis*). Even though only a small number of babies exposed to GBS develop infection, those who become infected can be seriously ill, with rapid progression to severe breathing difficulty and shock.

There are 2 periods after birth when GBS infections typically occur: *early onset* refers to the first week of life, and *late-onset* GBS typically occurs at 3 to 4 weeks of age, although late-onset GBS infection can occur anytime between 7 days and 3 months of age. Early-onset GBS is best prevented by giving antibiotics during labor to mothers who have a positive GBS screening test result. Late-onset GBS infection cannot be prevented but may be suspected as the cause when a baby shows signs of infection.

Central Line–Associated Bloodstream Infection

Central line–associated bloodstream infection (*CLABSI*) is a term used to describe a bacterial infection in the bloodstream of a baby who has a catheter placed in a major blood vessel (*central line*). These lines are frequently used in the NICU and include umbilical catheters and peripherally inserted central catheters (*PICC* lines). The most common bacteria causing CLABSI are *staphylococci* that normally live on the baby's skin. Most babies with CLABSI do not develop sudden or extreme signs of infection. Instead, they may gradually have more episodes of apnea or feeding problems. Sometimes, parents and caregivers say, "He just isn't acting right today."

At times, it can be difficult to determine if a baby truly has CLABSI because some staphylococcal bacteria always live on a baby's skin and can contaminate the blood culture bottle, resulting in a false-positive blood culture test result. On the other hand, the blood culture test result may be negative, but the baby appears to truly have an infection. The NICU team must use their best judgment to determine which newborns need treatment and for how long.

The health care team works hard to prevent CLABSI. Good hand washing, strict sterile methods during insertion of lines, expert care during use, and removing catheters as soon as they are no longer needed are key to preventing infections. Central line–associated bloodstream infections are treated with IV antibiotics. Frequently, central lines must be removed to successfully treat the infection. Although most newborns recover from the infection, it is a setback in their progress and often increases the length of their hospital stay.

> ❝ There's a lot of art in medicine, and sometimes different attending doctors will have different ideas about what's going on and how to address it. ❞
>
> Alex, father of **Pascal**

Preventing Hospital-Acquired Infections

Each NICU has its own policies for preventing infection. Your baby's nurse will tell you what to expect in your NICU. *Hand washing is the best way to protect your baby from a hospital-acquired infection.* Each time you come to the NICU, you will be asked to scrub your hands. Many NICUs supply alcohol hand gel at each bedside to use before and after touching your baby. If you or

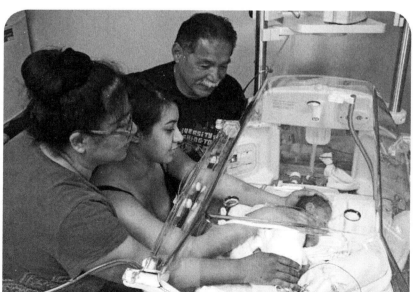

your family members have any signs of illness, consult your baby's doctor or nurse before coming to the NICU. In some cases, it may be better to stay away and get well rather than risk exposing your baby. What is a simple cold or stomach bug for you can become a very serious infection for your baby.

When your baby faces challenges, it may help to support each other as a family.
Courtesy of University of Washington Medical Center, Seattle, WA.

Problems With a Baby's Blood

Hypoglycemia

Hypoglycemia means *low blood sugar*. Your baby uses sugar (*glucose*) to produce energy. Before birth, mothers provide their fetus with a constant supply of glucose across the placenta. The fetus uses this glucose for energy and growth. During the last 3 months of pregnancy, healthy, full-term fetuses have the chance to store some glucose for use after birth. If the placenta was not working well, the fetus has not grown well, or the baby was born early, there may not be much glucose storage.

When the umbilical cord is cut, the glucose supply from the mother ends and the newborn has to depend on stored glucose or nutrients provided from breast milk, formula, or IV fluid. In healthy, full-term newborns, the blood glucose level falls during the first few hours after birth and then stabilizes as their body forms glucose from substances like protein and fat.

Risk of Hypoglycemia

Babies can become hypoglycemic for several reasons. Newborns of mothers with diabetes temporarily make too much of the hormone that lowers blood sugar (*insulin*). Babies who need resuscitation, become very cold, are working hard to breathe, or are born preterm or small for their gestational age can quickly use up whatever stored glucose they had resulting in hypoglycemia.

Signs of Hypoglycemia

The common signs of hypoglycemia include tremors or jitters, irregular breathing, and floppy muscle tone. Some newborns may not have any signs, so any baby who is at risk for hypoglycemia is carefully monitored. The fastest method is to test a drop of blood from the baby's heel, using a small glucose monitor at the baby's bedside. If the test result indicates low blood sugar, an additional sample may be sent to the laboratory for a more precise result.

Treatment of Hypoglycemia

Babies at risk of hypoglycemia and those who have mild, transient hypoglycemia may only need early and frequent feedings. If hypoglycemia is more significant, causes serious signs, or is persistent, it will be treated with IV fluids. Some babies have persistent, severe hypoglycemia and may need to have an IV line placed in a large blood vessel (such as an *umbilical venous catheter*) and receive IV fluids with a high concentration of sugar. Other babies may need to receive medications to raise their blood sugar and will have additional blood tests to diagnose the cause of the hypoglycemia.

Jaundice

Red blood cells (*RBCs*) have a short life span. When the body breaks down old blood cells, a substance called *bilirubin* is released into the bloodstream. Before the body can dispose of the bilirubin, the liver must change the bilirubin's chemical structure so it can be removed from the baby's body in his urine and bowel movements.

The enzyme in the baby's liver that causes this change is not very active at birth. In other words, it takes a few days to "turn on." Until the liver can do this job, bilirubin builds up in the newborn's blood and can be seen in the baby's skin as yellow skin color (*jaundice*).

Physiologic Jaundice

In most babies, bilirubin levels reach their peak toward the end of the first week and then gradually fall over the next 1 to 2 weeks. The peak level is higher in preterm newborns and may remain higher for longer. This type of jaundice is very common, occurring in nearly half of full-term newborns and up to 80% of preterm newborns. It does not mean that something is wrong with your baby's liver. It is simply a result of your baby's immature liver function and is called *physiologic jaundice.* Physiologic jaundice does not require any treatment.

Hyperbilirubinemia

If the bilirubin level rises higher or faster than normal, the condition is called *hyperbilirubinemia.* Some families have an inherited blood problem that causes higher bilirubin levels. Other problems, such as infection, may alter liver function and cause a rapid increase in bilirubin levels. If your baby is at risk for hyperbilirubinemia, his bilirubin levels will be monitored.

Anything that causes more RBCs to break down, such as bruising during birth, increases the amount of bilirubin the liver must handle. Blood type incompatibility between the mother and baby is another cause of increased RBC breakdown. (See Chapter 1.) If your baby is not feeding, he may have trouble eliminating the bilirubin from his body through bowel movements.

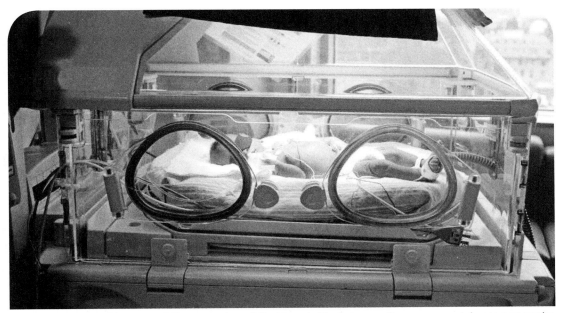

Phototherapy uses a blue-green light to treat hyperbilirubinemia. The baby usually wears eye patches to protect the eyes from the light.

Treatment of Hyperbilirubinemia

If the bilirubin level reaches a point that requires treatment, *phototherapy* will be started. Phototherapy uses blue-green light waves to change the shape of the bilirubin molecule so it can be eliminated in the baby's urine or stool without requiring the extra step in the liver. Patches are commonly placed over a baby's eyes during phototherapy to shield them from the bright light. Most newborns who require treatment for hyperbilirubinemia can be successfully treated with phototherapy. Rarely, phototherapy cannot adequately control the bilirubin level. In this case, an *exchange transfusion* may be necessary. During this procedure, a calculated amount of the baby's blood is withdrawn through an IV line in the umbilical cord (*umbilical catheter*) and replaced with matched blood from the blood bank.

With proper management, hyperbilirubinemia causes no long-term effects. The main reason hyperbilirubinemia is treated is because bilirubin is a molecule that can cross the brain's protective barrier. If excessively high levels of bilirubin pass into the brain, it can cause a disorder called *kernicterus* and result in brain damage. Kernicterus is a very rare problem in the United States.

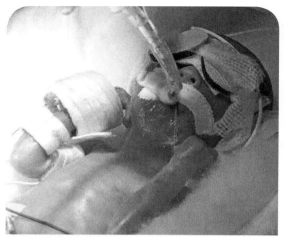

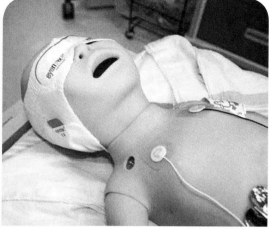

Holland wears eye patches that protect her eyes from the phototherapy lights.

The training manikin wears a different style of eye protection for phototherapy.

A Different Type of Jaundice

The common type of jaundice described previously is caused by *unconjugated bilirubin,* also called *indirect bilirubin.* A different type of jaundice is caused by *conjugated* or *direct bilirubin.* This is much less common and the causes are more complex. This type of hyperbilirubinemia often indicates an abnormality in liver function or a blockage in the flow of waste products leaving the liver. If your baby has conjugated hyperbilirubinemia, talk with your medical team to discuss the possible cause and treatment. Phototherapy does not help this type of hyperbilirubinemia.

Neurologic Problems

Birth Depression

If blood flow into or out of the placenta is decreased during labor, the fetus may not receive enough oxygen from the mother. When this happens, the fetal heart may have trouble pumping and it may not be able to provide enough blood flow and oxygen to other cells in the body. The baby may be born limp, not breathing, and with a low heart rate. This is called *birth depression.*

The lack of blood flow in the fetus is known as *ischemia.* The cells have low oxygen (the cells are *hypoxic*), cannot work properly, and begin to produce waste products in the form of acids. These acids build up, a condition called *acidemia,* and can damage many of the body's cells.

If birth depression from lack of blood flow and oxygen results in abnormal brain function, the condition is called *hypoxic-ischemic encephalopathy* (*HIE*).

Causes of Birth Depression

Anything that interferes with blood and oxygen flowing into or out of the placenta can cause birth depression. Problems with placental blood flow can occur because of infection, abnormal placental development, separation of the placenta from the uterus before birth, or a placenta that is not working well. All of these things can influence oxygen supply to the fetus.

The oxygen supply to the fetus is temporarily decreased during labor contractions; this is a normal and expected part of the labor process. However, sometimes, the mother has unusually strong contractions, contractions that are too close together, or contractions that each last an unusually long time. The umbilical cord carries blood and oxygen to the baby from the placenta and it can become squeezed during contractions if it is wrapped tightly around the baby, during a very difficult delivery, or if it slips into the birth canal before the baby (*prolapsed cord*).

Factors That Can Cause Birth Depression

- Separation of the placenta from the uterine wall before birth (*placental abruption*)
- Squeezing (*compression*) of the umbilical cord during labor and delivery, a cord tightened around the baby's neck (*nuchal cord*), a cord trapped below the baby in the birth canal (*prolapsed cord*)
- Prolonged or difficult delivery
- Unusual presentation during vaginal birth, such as buttocks first or legs first (*breech presentation*)
- Life-threatening maternal or fetal infection
- Maternal high blood pressure or severe low blood pressure (as in shock)
- Lack of oxygen to the mother (for example, due to acute asthma, severe pneumonia, or seizures)
- Umbilical cord accident (for example, a cord that ties in a knot in the uterus, a cord that tangles with a twin)
- Severe injury to the mother (for example, from a car crash)
- Severe lack of red blood cells (*anemia*) of the fetus due to infection, damage to the red blood cells, or bleeding into the mother's circulation or into a twin

Preventing Birth Depression

The obstetric team will try to identify pregnancies at risk for problems with placental function and help before the baby is affected. If the mother has high blood pressure or diabetes, for example, or if the fetus is not growing or gaining weight, prenatal testing with ultrasounds or electronic monitoring of the baby's heart rate may be done to make sure the fetus is in good condition. Labor may be induced or cesarean birth planned if the obstetric team decides that waiting for labor to start on its own could endanger the baby. During labor and delivery, fetal heart rate monitoring is one tool that can help detect problems. The goal is to deliver the baby before problems from poor placental function occur but not so early as to cause major problems of prematurity.

Severe birth depression is an unusual problem, with most factors being outside anyone's control. Birth depression is often unknown until a pregnant woman presents with a problem such as decreased fetal movement or continuous severe belly pain. During the mother's examination, the nurse or physician may detect a fetal heart rate that is too fast (*tachycardic*), too slow (*bradycardic*), or too steady (does not change in response to fetal movement or stimulation). The nurse or physician may find significant vaginal bleeding, abdominal tenderness, the umbilical cord in the birth canal (*prolapsed umbilical cord*), or other signs of potential fetal distress, like the presence of meconium (baby's first stool) in the amniotic fluid (see Meconium Aspiration Syndrome [MAS] earlier in this chapter).

Mild Birth Depression

Babies who have only mild birth depression may recover quickly after birth. The NICU team may need to provide breathing support for several minutes until the baby begins to breathe well on his own. After stabilization, babies with mild depression will be monitored. Sometimes, feeding will be delayed to allow the bowel to rest and recover from a possible interruption in adequate oxygen.

Severe Birth Depression

Babies with severe birth depression may need a more complex resuscitation. The NICU team may need to place a temporary breathing tube in his windpipe (*endotracheal intubation*), do chest compressions, and give emergency fluids and medications.

Newborns with severe birth depression often need help breathing with a ventilator. Occasionally, the blood vessels in the lungs don't relax properly, leading to a condition called PPHN (see Persistent Pulmonary Hypertension of the Newborn [PPHN] earlier in this chapter). They may have decreased heart function and need medications to help their heart pump with more strength. They need very careful management of glucose and fluids, especially if the kidneys have been injured by lack of blood flow and oxygen. Brain injury often leads to seizures during the first days of life. Babies with severe birth depression are often very ill and have major complications, and some do not survive.

Complications of Birth Depression

- Seizures
- Brain injury
- Low blood pressure
- Respiratory distress
- Kidney injury
- Bowel injury
- Low blood sugar
- Bleeding

Hypoxic-ischemic Encephalopathy

Birth depression can result in HIE. As described earlier, HIE is caused by lack of oxygen in the blood (*hypoxia*) and reduced blood flow to the brain (*ischemia*). These events lead to brain dysfunction (*encephalopathy*).

Hypoxic-ischemic encephalopathy is often divided into 3 stages: mild, moderate, and severe. Most often, mild HIE has a good outcome and treatment in the newborn period is only supportive, as described previously. Moderate and severe HIE continue to be important causes of acute brain injury and may benefit from additional therapy.

Therapeutic Hypothermia

Therapeutic hypothermia, also called *cooling*, is a safe and effective treatment for term and near-term babies with moderate or severe HIE. Lowering the baby's body temperature after birth appears to reduce the amount of damage to brain cells and improve the chance of survival without major disabilities. It appears to be most effective for babies with moderate HIE but is also offered to babies with more severe HIE.

Babies must meet certain conditions to qualify for therapeutic hypothermia, and it appears to be most effective if it is started within the first few hours after birth. Therapeutic hypothermia is provided in specialized NICUs. This often requires rapid transport of eligible babies so cooling can be started in time.

The 2 methods currently being used are *selective head cooling* and *whole body cooling*. For selective head cooling, the baby wears a special cooling cap. For whole body cooling, the baby lays on a cooling mattress. With either method, the baby's rectal temperature is kept at about 34.5°C (94°F) for 72 hours. The baby's heart rate often decreases, but as long as the blood pressure and oxygen saturation are stable, no assistance is needed. At the end of the cooling period, the baby is gradually rewarmed.

Outcome for Babies With Birth Depression

Most babies recover well from mild or moderate birth depression, but some will have long-term disabilities, such as problems thinking, seeing, hearing, or walking. Even with hypothermia treatment, many newborns with severe HIE will die or survive with disabilities. It may be very difficult for doctors to predict how well your baby will do until months or even years later. Sometimes, brain imaging in the newborn period using magnetic resonance imaging (*MRI*) can provide some clues about the baby's likelihood of having disabilities.

Seizures

Seizures occur when there is a sudden surge of electrical signals in the brain. Seizures can be a sign of brain injury or irritation. They may appear as jerking movements of the arms or legs, stiffening of an extremity or arching of the back, facial twitching, head turning, or repetitive movements of the eyes, lips, or tongue. A pause in breathing (*apnea*) and sudden increases in blood pressure may also occur. At times, seizures can be very subtle and hard to detect. Babies can have normal jittery movements that are not seizures. Normal jittery movements stop when a hand is placed on the baby's trembling arms or legs, however; seizure activity does not.

Causes of Seizures

Often, no cause can be found. Seizures may result from brain injury, infection, chemical imbalances in the blood (for example, low blood sugar, low calcium), bleeding in the brain or surrounding tissues, swelling of the brain, or malformation of the brain.

Diagnosis of Seizures

If the NICU team suspects seizures, they will study your baby's brain waves using a cerebral function monitor (see Chapter 3) or a painless test called an *electroencephalogram* (*EEG*). This test involves placing sensors on the baby's scalp and recording the electrical activity in the baby's brain. Seizures appear as abnormal patterns of electrical activity on the brain-wave tracing.

Other tests that may be done include

- An ultrasound of the brain to look for bleeding or unusual brain structure
- Computed tomography (*CT*) scan or MRI to look for bleeding, swelling, or unusual brain structure or unusual blood vessels
- Blood tests to look for chemical imbalances (for example, glucose, sodium, calcium, acids)
- Blood and spinal fluid tests to look for infection

A doctor specializing in disorders of the brain and nervous system (*neurologist*) may also examine your baby and help the NICU team manage your baby's problems.

Treatment for Seizures

The first priority is to treat any underlying cause of the seizure, such as low blood sugar. Seizures are treated with medications that decrease the brain's electrical activity. The duration of treatment varies from just a few days to several months or longer, depending on the underlying problem and frequency of seizures.

Potential Outcome for a Baby With Seizures

The outcome for a baby who has seizures depends on what is causing the seizures, presence of brain injury from the underlying cause, severity of seizures, and type of seizures. Many babies recover completely, with no signs of brain damage, especially if the seizures are brief and infrequent. Seizures caused by severe birth depression or serious brain injury may persist for a longer period and have a higher risk of resulting in learning disabilities, developmental delays, and neurologic abnormalities. Follow-up visits with the neurologist or developmental specialists may be needed to evaluate your baby's progress over a long period.

Stay Informed

This chapter has explained many of the serious medical problems that can bring a baby to the NICU. This information is intended to give you a basic understanding of each problem but does not replace discussions with your baby's NICU team.

Keep in mind that just as each baby is unique, so is each NICU. There are different approaches to treating many of these problems, and new discoveries are helping to improve the care of babies every day.

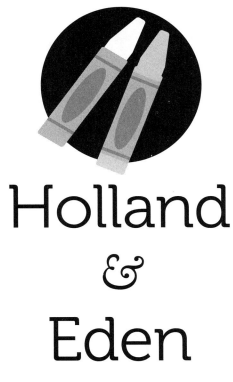

Holland

&

Eden

Born at 24 weeks 3 days

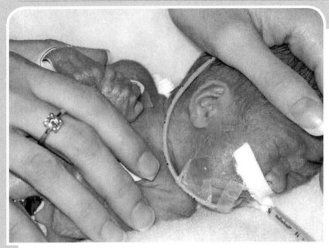

Mom's hands comfort Holland.

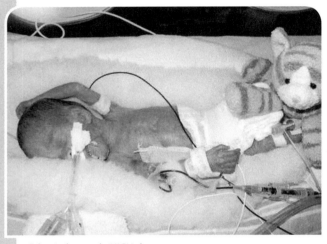

Eden in her early NICU days.

Holland and Eden were born at 24 weeks 3 days' gestation, weighing just over 1 pound each. At the time of their birth, there was no infection, no abnormalities, and never an explanation for why they came so early. They were born with their eyes still fused shut and skin so thin that you could see through it. They were perfectly formed and, to us, already beautiful.

Our girls spent the first 110 days of their lives in the NICU. During that time, we had some very long and very sad days. Both girls were transferred for patent ductus arteriosus (PDA) ligation surgery on their hearts. They both underwent laser surgery on their eyes for retinopathy of prematurity. We lived through more than one infection, one which Holland almost didn't survive. Both had some degree of bleeding in the brain. Both needed a lot of coaxing to learn to eat and grow. We experienced a great deal of guilt, grief, and devastation.

Our time in the NICU was also filled with small moments of happiness and even times of great joy. I clearly remember the nurse who asked if I wanted to hold each baby for the first time and how much work they would do to get us ready for kangaroo care. I remember the care with which they taught us how to touch our babies, how to change their tiny diapers, how to take their temperatures. I remember the doctors giving hugs and high fives when Holland's platelets finally went back up following a nasty infection. I remember them listening to our endless questions and sitting down with us to draw diagrams to help us understand complicated medical issues, never annoyed by our incessant attention to detail. I remember the encouragement they gave me in pumping and attempting to breastfeed and how they kept me motivated by always oohing and aahing over the calorie content of my milk. I will be forever grateful to the doctors and nurses who touched our lives at that time and took such good care of our family.

Unfortunately, our struggles did not end when we left the NICU. We went home with oxygen, and monitors, and countless doctor appointments for the first 6 months. Holland has had ongoing issues with asthma, vision, mild cerebral palsy (CP), attention, and anxiety. She has had multiple eye surgeries and has been hospitalized several times with pneumonia and respiratory illnesses. She did not start walking until after she was 2, and still struggles to keep up with her peers in physical activities. Eating and growing continue to be a challenge, and she did not hit 50 pounds until this past summer.

Eden has more severe CP and is unable to stand or walk. She uses a power wheelchair as her main source of mobility. We spend a lot of time and money on equipment and therapies to help her achieve her potential. In addition to the CP, Eden was diagnosed with profound bilateral hearing loss at 6 months of age and underwent her first cochlear implant surgery when she was 14 months old. She received her second implant in 2014 at age 9. She also underwent vocal cord reinnervation surgery in 2014 to help improve her vocal quality from a paralyzed vocal cord. Between the 2 girls, we have been through 12 surgeries.

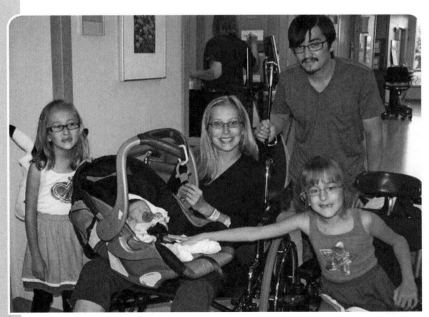

A take-home baby! Violet was born in 2012.

While I feel like it is important for people to be aware of the ongoing issues that extremely premature infants face, I really hate listing their disabilities or medical issues when describing them. Terms like "chronic lung disease," or "profound hearing loss," or "cerebral palsy" do not give you any insight into the amazing people that they are becoming. I'd rather tell you about how Eden's smile lights up a room and how Holland's giggles are completely contagious. They are in fifth grade at our neighborhood school and are both voracious readers. Holland is passionate about video games, Pokémon, Skylanders, and stand-up comedy. She loves stories of all kinds and still loves to pretend. She also loves exploring nature, swimming, and collecting trinkets.

Eden loves adventure, from snorkeling to roller coasters to big cities, and pictures herself traveling the world, next stop…Tokyo. She loves Japanese manga and learning about Asian culture. She is a blossoming foodie who will try anything and shares her Dad's appetite for spicy mussels. She also loves having big discussions about everything from health care to history, world religions to disability rights. They both enrich our lives and bring us such joy every day.

I am not a person who believes that everything happens for a reason. What I *do* believe is that when bad things happen, we can become better people because of them. We can learn and grow from them. I am a better person because of my kids and what they have gone through following their traumatic birth. I do not take life for granted. I don't sweat the small stuff. I have learned to appreciate every step of progress they make, no matter how small it may seem. I am better able to support people who are going through similar circumstances. I am more compassionate and a better advocate for my children's needs. In addition to all of that, I have had the opportunity to meet so many incredible people who I would never have known otherwise, and my life is richer because of them.

Billie, mother of Holland and Eden

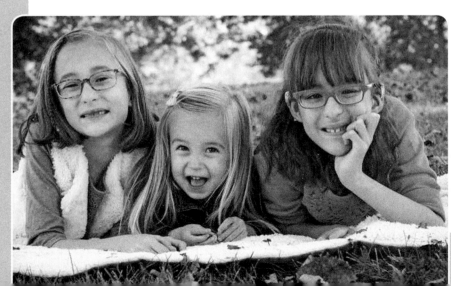

Holland, Violet, and Eden.

CHAPTER 5

Your Preterm Baby

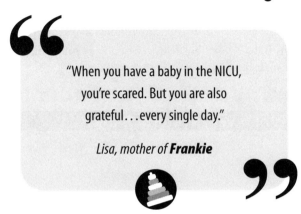

"When you have a baby in the NICU, you're scared. But you are also grateful...every single day."

*Lisa, mother of **Frankie***

More than 380,000 babies are born prematurely (preterm) in the United States each year. While the rate of preterm birth has been decreasing, we still expect about 1 in 10 babies in the United States to be born too soon. Preterm birth can be related to problems with the mother's health or a problem with the growing fetus, but about half the time, preterm labor happens for unknown reasons.

By the time your baby is born, even if she is born very early, all the major body systems have been formed, but they are immature and still developing. The organ systems may not function the same way they would in a full-term newborn and are at risk of injury or abnormal development.

Your baby's neonatal intensive care unit (NICU) team knows the wide range of problems that can affect preterm newborns. They can recognize early signs of developing problems and take steps that keep little problems from becoming a major crisis. Keep in mind that even though a baby is *at risk* of developing a problem, it does not mean that she *will* develop the problem. Talk with your NICU team about any concerns you have for your preterm baby.

How Does a Preterm Baby Look?

Your baby's appearance is related to her gestational age at birth. In fact, by examining your baby's physical features, the NICU team can estimate your baby's gestational age within a couple of weeks. This examination is called a *Ballard score*. The information listed below in the box titled "Physical Features of a Very Preterm Baby" describes features of a very preterm baby. Babies who are more mature will have fewer of these features.

Physical Features of a Very Preterm Baby

- Fused (closed) eyelids
- Thin, smooth skin
- Visible veins under the skin, especially over the tummy
- Flat or invisible nipples
- No fine hair (*lanugo*) over the baby's back and neck
- Smooth soles of the feet
- Soft, thin ears that do not spring back when folded
- No testes yet positioned in the scrotum (boys)
- Little fat in the vaginal labia (girls)
- Flexible joints at the hips and knees
- Limp muscle tone

Why Are Preterm Babies at Greater Risk of Complications?

The more preterm a baby is, the higher her risk of complications and the higher the level of care she will likely need. Preterm babies are more at risk because they are born with

- Immature lungs and a decreased amount of *surfactant,* a slippery soap-like substance that keeps the tiny air sacs in the lungs from collapsing as the baby breathes in and out

- Weak muscles that make it difficult to breathe

- Thin skin and reduced fat that puts the baby at risk for a low body temperature (*hypothermia*)

- Immature tissues that are easily damaged if exposed to too much oxygen

- Immature immune system that puts the baby at risk of infection

- Immature blood vessels in the brain that are easily damaged and bleed

▪ Less stored glucose that puts the baby at risk for low blood sugar (*hypoglycemia*)

▪ Smaller blood volume that puts the baby at risk for reduced number of red blood cells (*anemia*)

Problems Affecting the Preterm Baby's Lungs

The lungs are responsible for maintaining the correct amount of oxygen and carbon dioxide in your baby's body. Too much or too little of either gas is not healthy.

When you breathe in, air travels into the lungs through a series of tubes that gradually get smaller until air reaches tiny sacs called *alveoli*. In the alveoli, oxygen moves into the bloodstream to be carried to the rest of the body. Carbon dioxide is brought to the lungs through the bloodstream and moves into the alveoli to be exhaled when you breathe out.

Preterm babies may have difficulty with many of the lung's functions. These problems may begin in the delivery room and include difficulty beginning the process of breathing, keeping their lungs open, and controlling their breathing rate.

Breathing Problems at Birth

Before delivery, a baby's lungs are full of fluid and do not provide oxygen to the body. Instead, oxygen moves from the mother's blood through the placenta to the fetus. At birth, babies must quickly remove the fluid from their lungs, begin breathing, inflate their lungs with air, and use their lungs to carry oxygen to the blood.

Although many preterm babies will cry at birth and require little help from the NICU team, more than half of babies delivered before 33 weeks' gestation will have trouble breathing. The health care professional caring for your baby at birth may use a face mask and mechanical device to assist your baby's first breaths. Babies born very preterm may need to have a breathing tube placed in their throat and advanced to their windpipe (*endotracheal intubation*) to provide more assistance with breathing.

> 66 He was having a lot of trouble breathing on his own, so he was going to be intubated. It was that exact moment that I realized how serious this whole situation was. That moment defined me as a new mom of a preemie. 99
>
> Marnie, mother of **Kellan**

Respiratory Distress Syndrome (RDS)

Respiratory distress syndrome (RDS) is the most common lung condition affecting preterm babies. It mostly affects babies born before 35 weeks' gestation, but more mature newborns can develop RDS. The earlier a baby is born, the more likely she is to have RDS, and the more severe the disease is likely to be.

Respiratory distress syndrome is caused by immaturity of the baby's chest and lungs and a decreased amount of *surfactant*. Surfactant is a soap-like substance made in the lungs that coats the inside of the tiny breathing sacs (*alveoli*) and helps to keep them open as the baby breathes in and out. Without enough surfactant, the alveoli tend to collapse between breaths. If the alveoli collapse, the baby has to do extra work to reopen them with each breath. Over time, the oxygen level may decrease and the carbon dioxide level may increase in the baby's blood.

Each baby's lungs mature at a different rate. Surfactant production begins around the 24th week of gestation, but the system is not fully developed until 34 to 36 weeks. Giving steroids to the mother before a preterm delivery is safe for the mother and her fetus and can help speed up the production of surfactant in the fetal lungs.

Signs of RDS

Preterm babies may show signs of RDS within minutes after birth, or they may develop breathing problems in the first few hours after birth. You may notice your baby is breathing fast (*tachypnea*) or working hard to breathe. She may have labored breathing that causes the skin and muscles between the ribs or just below the rib cage to pull in during breaths (*retractions*) or grunting (a moaning sound) when she breathes out. Your baby may have a blue color around her lips called *cyanosis* or a pale and blotchy (*mottled*) appearance to her skin. If your baby is working hard to breathe and gets tired, her breathing rate may become uneven and she may take pauses in her breathing, called *apnea*.

> 66 You don't realize how strong you have to be to be a preemie parent, a NICU parent. These babies give us the emotional ride of our lives. 99
>
> Lisa, mother of **Frankie**

Auggie follows a fairly typical pathway through respiratory support devices.

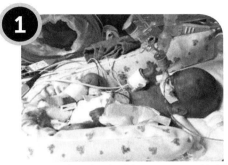

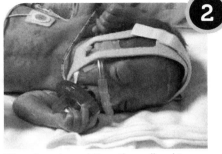

For several weeks after his very preterm birth, **Auggie** needed endotracheal intubation and a ventilator to help him breathe. Not all preterm babies need a ventilator after birth.

When **Auggie** could breathe well on his own, he used a nasal cannula to deliver CPAP to lessen the work of breathing.

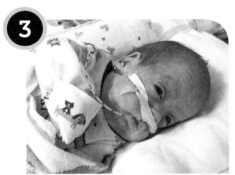

When **Auggie** grew stronger, he graduated from CPAP and used a nasal cannula to provide a gentle flow of air/oxygen.

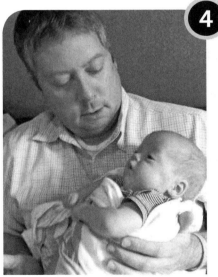

Finallly, **Auggie** no longer needed extra air flow or oxygen through the nasal cannula and is shown here with his proud father.

Diagnosis of RDS

If RDS is suspected, your baby's team may order a chest x-ray (*radiograph*) and a laboratory test called a *blood gas*. Babies with RDS often have a hazy white and grainy look to their chest radiograph. Their blood gas results may show a low oxygen level and a high carbon dioxide level. There is, however, no perfect test to diagnose RDS. The radiograph of a newborn with RDS looks a lot like a radiograph of a newborn with pneumonia. Respiratory distress syndrome is diagnosed by studying the radiographic findings and blood test results in combination with the baby's history, physical examination, and progress over the first days of life.

Treatment of RDS: Continuous Positive Airway Pressure (CPAP) and Surfactant

The best options for treating RDS continue to be an area of active research. Babies with mild RDS may only require additional oxygen through small plastic prongs called a *nasal cannula*.

If the baby has more serious RDS, she may receive oxygen and breathing support through CPAP. Nasal CPAP provides a constant low pressure of air (and sometimes, supplemental oxygen) into the baby's lungs through prongs placed in the nose or through a small mask placed over the nose. (See Chapter 3.) Nasal CPAP helps to stabilize the alveoli and prevent them from collapsing between breaths. Although CPAP helps to keep the baby's lungs open, the machine does not provide any breaths, so the baby has to breathe on her own.

Babies with the most serious RDS may need additional surfactant administered into their lungs and breathing assistance from a mechanical ventilator while their lungs mature. If mechanical ventilation is needed, a breathing tube (*endotracheal tube*) is temporarily placed in the baby's windpipe (*trachea*) in a procedure called *intubation*. (See Chapter 1.)

Frequently, preterm babies with respiratory distress are treated with CPAP first. If the baby has worsening difficulty breathing, the baby is intubated and surfactant is given through the breathing tube. Sometimes, the endotracheal tube is removed immediately after surfactant is administered, and the baby is given another chance on CPAP. Sometimes, the baby needs to stay intubated and receive breathing support from a ventilator for a period. Depending on the baby's response, 1 or 2 more doses of surfactant may be given. The goal is to decrease the amount of additional oxygen needed and the time spent on the ventilator.

If your baby will be born preterm, ask a member of the NICU team what you can expect regarding CPAP and surfactant.

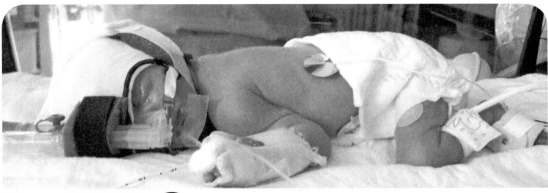

Allison needed CPAP at birth.

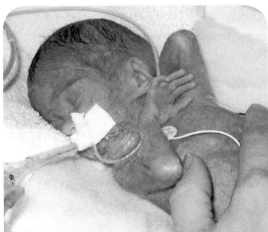

Eden needed intubation and a ventilator to help her breathe.

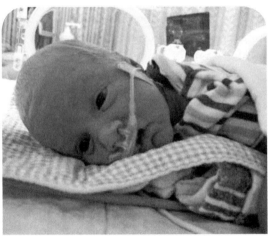

At 4 days old, **Reece** no longer needed the steady airway pressure from CPAP and graduated to a nasal cannula with a gentle flow of air/oxygen only.

Air Leaks

Air leaks were described in Chapter 4. They occur when breathing sacs (*alveoli*) rupture, allowing air to leak into the tissue surrounding the lung. Preterm babies are at higher risk for air leaks because babies with RDS have stiff lungs that don't open and close as easily as healthy lungs. When a baby with stiff lungs breathes or receives help from CPAP or a ventilator, one or more of the thin-walled alveoli can rupture. In preterm babies with RDS, surfactant helps decrease the risk of air leaks. If air becomes trapped between the lung and rib cage (*pneumothorax*), the air may be removed with a needle or a vacuum system attached to a thin plastic or silicone tube (*chest tube*).

Pulmonary interstitial emphysema (*PIE*) is a special type of air leak in which air becomes trapped in many small spaces and cannot be removed. Babies with PIE often require gentle ventilator support until their lungs heal. The NICU team may allow the baby to have lower blood oxygen levels or higher carbon dioxide levels temporarily to decrease the ventilator pressure while the lungs are healing. In some cases, a special ventilator (*high frequency ventilator*) that delivers tiny breaths at a high rate of speed may be used (see Chapter 4).

Bronchopulmonary Dysplasia (BPD)

Bronchopulmonary dysplasia (*BPD*) is a lung disease occurring mostly in babies born between 23 and 32 weeks' gestation. It may also be called *chronic lung disease* or *CLD*. The definition of BPD varies but is often described as a preterm baby born at less than 32 weeks' gestation who has required additional oxygen (more than 21% oxygen) for at least 4 weeks and continues to require oxygen when she becomes what would have been 36 weeks' gestational age.

Researchers are still trying to understand exactly what causes BPD and how it can be prevented. Babies with BPD have fewer, larger alveoli and fewer blood vessels surrounding their alveoli. This means the lungs have a smaller area to use for breathing. In addition, some babies with BPD may have thickened, swollen, and scarred airways within their lungs. This damage might be caused by mechanical injury and inflammation from repeated opening and closing of the tiny alveoli. Inflammation is part of the body's response to an injury and can promote healing, but when inflammation gets out of control, it can damage the body.

Risk Factors for BPD

Researchers still do not know why some preterm babies without any risk factors get BPD. Genetics and family history may play a role because inherited genes can affect how your baby's lungs respond to an injury.

Overall, BPD occurs in approximately 20% of babies who are born before 30 weeks' gestation, but the rate of BPD varies widely among different hospitals. Some of the risk factors for BPD are listed below in the box titled "Risk Factors for Bronchopulmonary Dysplasia."

Risk Factors for Bronchopulmonary Dysplasia

- Lower gestational age at birth
- Infection of the amniotic fluid before birth (*chorioamnionitis*)
- Severe respiratory distress syndrome (*RDS*)
- Prolonged mechanical ventilation
- Pneumonia
- Poor nutrition
- Excess fluid in the lung

Diagnosis and Treatment of BPD

Babies with RDS usually begin to improve after several days to a week of treatment. Newborns who develop BPD often have more severe RDS at first, are slow to improve, or may begin to improve and then stop making progress. Chest radiographs may show a hazy, streaky, or bubbly appearance in the lungs.

The goal of BPD treatment is to allow the newborn's lung to heal while new, undamaged lung tissue develops. Treatment for BPD includes providing additional oxygen as needed, providing good nutrition with enough calories to promote growth, and avoiding excess fluid in the lungs. Additional vitamin A in your baby's diet may help prevent BPD. Other medications may be used to help improve your baby's lung function, but none have been proven to prevent BPD or change its course. Medications like furosemide (Lasix), spironolactone (Aldactone), and chlorothiazide (Diuril) help babies make additional urine and may also help decrease the amount of fluid in the lungs. Babies with BPD may produce additional mucus and have episodes of wheezing or narrowing of the air passages (*bronchospasm*). If your baby has episodes of wheezing, inhaled medications may help expand your baby's airway.

Some babies with BPD have sudden changes in vital signs, commonly called *spells,* especially when they become upset. During a spell, the baby may become blue (*cyanotic*), have a low heart rate (*bradycardia*), and have a lower oxygen level (*oxygen desaturation* or *desat*). Sometimes, spells occur at a predictable time each day. Parents and caregivers can often identify the triggers that begin these episodes and learn how to prevent or stop them.

Babies with the most severe BPD may require treatment with a steroid to decrease the inflammation in their lungs. Although steroids given to mothers before preterm birth are safe and helpful, steroids are not routinely given to preterm babies after birth. They may offer short-term benefits by allowing babies to wean off of a mechanical ventilator earlier; however, they may interfere with normal brain development and increase the risk of long-term disabilities. Because of this possible risk, health care professionals currently avoid giving babies steroids after preterm birth except in severe cases of respiratory failure.

Complications of BPD

Bronchopulmonary dysplasia is different for every baby. Many babies who need help breathing will have mild or moderate BPD. Mild BPD can mean that your baby requires oxygen for a month or longer but is able to go home without extra oxygen or medications. Babies with moderate BPD may need to go home with oxygen for a time, and others may require home oxygen for several months. Babies with the most severe BPD may require a prolonged hospital stay and even a home ventilator program.

Babies with BPD often have difficulty feeding by mouth. They may develop a bad reaction to having things placed in their mouth, called *oral aversion*. Some babies with BPD may have slow emptying from their stomach, and feedings may flow backward into their food pipe (*esophagus*). This backward flow is called *reflux*. Physical or occupational therapists may help the NICU team develop a treatment plan for babies with BPD who have difficulty with feeding.

Bronchopulmonary dysplasia is a chronic disease that can take months or, occasionally, years to heal. Because your baby could miss the normal stages of infant growth, your baby's nurse or therapist will work with you and your baby on a variety of exercises and activities designed to promote your baby's best possible growth and development.

At birth, preterm babies only have a small number of the alveoli they will have when they are fully grown. The lungs continue to grow, and new alveoli develop for several years. Most babies with BPD show gradual improvement in their lung function after discharge but may have some abnormal lung function for years. They may not be able to deal with pollution in the air and should not be exposed to tobacco smoke. Babies with BPD have an increased risk of developing asthma and pneumonia. If they develop a respiratory infection like a cold or flu (*influenza*), they may become very ill and require rehospitalization. Before discharge, your baby may receive an injection (palivizumab [Synagis]) to help prevent complications from a common viral infection called RSV (*respiratory syncytial virus*) that occurs during the fall and winter. (See Chapter 8.) It is important for everyone who comes in contact with your baby to wash their hands and get a flu vaccination.

Apnea of Prematurity

Even though a fetus doesn't use her lungs for actual breathing, she does make breathing movements before birth. This breathing isn't continuous and doesn't have a regular pattern. After birth, babies must develop a regular breathing pattern, even when they are sleeping, to maintain a constant supply of oxygen. Breathing patterns are controlled by a timing mechanism in the baby's brain, and the timing mechanism is not fully mature until a baby is close to full term.

Preterm babies often have irregular, or uneven, breathing patterns with episodes of shallow breathing or pauses. A prolonged breathing pause is called *apnea*. Apnea is one of the most common problems of prematurity, occurring in 25% of all preterm babies and in more than 80% of babies weighing less than 1,000 g (about 2 lb 3 oz) at birth. Short pauses that occur several times in a row are called *periodic breathing*. This pattern is common, especially during sleep, even among healthy term babies, and may last for many weeks after birth.

When a preterm baby has apnea or becomes apneic, her heart rate may slow and her blood oxygen level may decrease. Slowing of the heart rate is called *bradycardia* (*brady* for short) and decreases in oxygen saturation are called *desaturations* (*desat* for short). The NICU team may call these events *As and Bs* for *apneas and bradycardias* or *A-B-Ds* for *apneas, bradycardias, and desaturations*.

Management of Apnea of Prematurity

Babies at risk for apnea have an electronic monitor that tracks their heart and breathing rates. They may also be monitored with a pulse oximeter to track the oxygen saturation in their blood. Alarms go off when the heart rate, breathing rate, or oxygen saturation falls below an acceptable level for a certain period.

> " The babies would just stop breathing and an alarm would go off and nurses would run in, jiggle the babies a little, and then they would breathe. That became normal for us, and it got to the point where the alarm would go off and by the time the nurses arrived, we had gotten them breathing again. "
>
> Bridget, mother of **Bailey Jo** and **Abraham**

Apnea can be very frightening for parents, but many apneic periods end on their own and the baby begins to breathe again. If the baby does not begin breathing on her own, the caregiver may gently rub the baby's side or foot to encourage breathing. Sometimes, the caregiver also needs to give the baby extra oxygen. If the baby doesn't start breathing after stimulation or the heart rate remains low, a caregiver may need to give several assisted breaths with a face mask. Babies with frequent apnea that leads to bradycardia and desaturation may require medication, CPAP, or extra airflow from a nasal cannula. *Caffeine* is a medicine, given intravenously or by mouth, that stimulates the brain's breathing center and may help to normalize the baby's breathing pattern.

As the baby matures, apnea of prematurity gradually improves and finally disappears. Apnea of prematurity resolves in most preterm babies before they go home. Once apnea of prematurity resolves, it does not come back. Very preterm babies, delivered before 28 weeks' gestation, may not have fully mature breathing control until several weeks after their due date. A small number of these babies may require home apnea monitoring after discharge.

Apnea of prematurity is not the same as sudden infant death syndrome (*SIDS*; also called crib death) and is not a risk factor for SIDS. The cause of SIDS is unknown. Strategies for reducing the risk of SIDS are found in Chapter 9.

Treatment Options for Apnea of Prematurity

- Careful monitoring until the baby outgrows apnea
- Caffeine
- CPAP or airflow from a nasal cannula

Obstructive Apnea

Obstructive apnea occurs when the baby is trying to breathe but the airway becomes blocked. Preterm babies have low muscle tone in the upper throat, making the airway more likely to become blocked. During sleep, the airway may partially collapse and block air movement into the lungs. Obstructive apnea may also occur while a baby is being fed or held if the head falls too far forward or backward and closes the airway.

Problems Affecting the Preterm Baby's Blood

Anemia

Anemia means there is a decrease in the number of red blood cells (*RBCs*) in a baby's blood. Red blood cells are the part of blood that carries oxygen. The NICU team often estimates the number of RBCs by a blood test that measures the *hemoglobin* level or *hematocrit*.

Causes of Anemia

Anemia is a common problem and has multiple causes. Preterm babies are at risk of anemia because their blood cells have a shorter life span and their body has a limited ability to make new blood cells. In total, a 1,500-g (3 lb 5 oz) baby has approximately 4 ounces of blood in her body. Blood may be lost during birth because of a problem with the placenta or umbilical cord, or internal bleeding may cause sudden, severe blood loss. During the first few weeks of life, blood may be lost if a baby requires frequent laboratory tests. A very common cause of anemia is a decrease in blood production called *anemia of prematurity*.

> The NICU is an amazing place where amazing medicine happens. It can also be an extremely lonely place. Without the empathy and compassion from the doctors and nurses, I'm not sure how anyone could survive those first few weeks.
>
> Amanda, mother of **Maxwell**

Anemia of Prematurity

Anemia of prematurity occurs because RBC production temporarily stops after birth. A hormone called *erythropoietin* (*EPO*) is made in your baby's liver and kidney. Erythropoietin stimulates RBC production in the baby's bone marrow. Shortly after birth, EPO production stops and the bone marrow stops making RBCs. The baby's hemoglobin level gradually decreases over several weeks, reaching its lowest value between 4 to 10 weeks after birth. Eventually, the hemoglobin reaches a level at which EPO is secreted again and RBC production resumes. This is a process that occurs even in full-term babies; however, it occurs earlier, lasts longer, and is more severe in preterm babies.

Diagnosis of Anemia

If anemia occurs very suddenly because of rapid blood loss, babies may have signs of shock, with low blood pressure, fast heart rate, weak pulses, pale or ashen gray skin color, and respiratory distress. Anemia of prematurity causes a more gradual decrease in RBCs and may cause no signs at all. Babies with anemia of prematurity may have a pale color to their skin and gums. They may have poor growth, decreased activity, a rapid heart rate, rapid breathing, an increase in apnea events, or feeding difficulties.

If the cause of anemia is not readily apparent, the NICU team may order diagnostic tests to look for evidence of bleeding or blood cell destruction. Babies with anemia of prematurity may have their hemoglobin level and hematocrit monitored regularly to ensure they do not fall too low. A blood test called the *reticulocyte count* may be checked intermittently to monitor how quickly the bone marrow is making new RBCs.

Treatment of Anemia of Prematurity

Babies without symptoms may not require any treatment. They may receive additional iron in their diet to ensure there is enough iron in their body to support RBC production once it begins. Some hospitals will give regular injections of EPO to prevent or treat anemia of prematurity; however, this treatment remains controversial and is not routinely practiced in the United States. Babies with symptomatic anemia may require one or more blood transfusions.

The likelihood of requiring a blood transfusion is related to the degree of prematurity at birth. The more preterm a baby is, and the more significant health problems a baby has, the greater the risk of requiring transfusions. There is no single rule for receiving a blood transfusion. Researchers continue to investigate the risks and benefits of different blood transfusion practices. Currently, more than half of babies born before 28 weeks' gestation will receive at least one blood transfusion.

> Take some time at the beginning of the NICU experience and get organized. Appoint a willing friend to coordinate your other friends who want to help with groceries, meal prep, house cleaning, yard work, walking the dog, etc. This will help you maintain your sanity and your energy.
>
> Lisa, mother of **Frankie**

Problems Affecting the Preterm Baby's Heart

Patent Ductus Arteriosus (PDA)

While in the womb, all healthy fetuses have a bridging artery that connects the 2 large blood vessels leaving the heart. This bridging artery is called the *ductus arteriosus.* Within a few days after a healthy term birth, the ductus arteriosus should close when the muscle surrounding the artery squeezes tightly. In preterm babies, the ductus arteriosus may remain open after birth or reopen in the weeks following birth. This is referred to as a *patent* (open) *ductus arteriosus* or *PDA*.

If the ductus arteriosus remains open, it may allow too much blood to enter the lungs and lead to heart and breathing problems. A PDA affects nearly half of babies born at less than 30 weeks' gestation or weighing less than 1,000 g (about 2 lb 3 oz). The more preterm a baby is at birth, the greater the risk of a PDA that causes trouble. The signs of a PDA often occur toward the end of the first week of life.

Signs of a PDA

The signs of a PDA depend on how widely open the ductus arteriosus is, how much blood is flowing through it, and the direction the blood is flowing. The signs of a PDA may include a *heart murmur,* breathing problems, an enlarged heart, feeding difficulties, or decreased urine output.

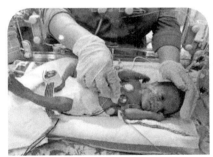

A heart murmur is a swooshing sound heard with a stethoscope. Heart murmurs are very common in newborns, sometimes come and go, and do not necessarily mean there is a problem. Sometimes, the largest PDAs have very soft murmurs or none at all, and very small PDAs may have loud murmurs. The signs of a PDA may vary over the course of several hours.

Listening with a stethoscope gives the nurse information about **Lucy's** heart and lungs.

Diagnosis of a PDA

If the NICU team suspects a PDA, an *echocardiogram* (*echo* for short) may be ordered. An echocardiogram is an ultrasound of the heart that can show if the ductus arteriosus is open. Echocardiograms use sound waves to create moving images. There is no radiation exposure from an echocardiogram.

Treatment of a PDA

The treatment of a PDA depends on its size and the amount of difficulty it is causing your baby. A small PDA in an otherwise healthy preterm baby may cause few problems and may not need treatment. Many small preterm babies, however, do not tolerate a PDA and will need treatment.

If medical treatment is required, *indomethacin, acetaminophen,* or *ibuprofen* may be given. These medications are given through an intravenous (IV) line and have similar functions. They interfere with a chemical in the body that relaxes the muscle surrounding the PDA. The goal is to make the muscle squeeze tightly, close the ductus, and, ultimately, cause it to "glue" shut. Each of the medications used to treat a PDA can affect kidney function. After receiving any of these medications, many babies will make less urine and retain water. This usually goes away in several days. Until it resolves, the NICU team may limit your baby's fluids.

If the medication does not work or can't be used because of other problems, surgery may be needed. When the surgery is over, there will be a bandage over the incision and possibly a chest tube to drain any bleeding. The chest tube is usually removed within a day or two after surgery. Some babies may be sicker after the surgery than they were before surgery. They may have trouble with low blood pressure or more significant breathing problems until they fully recover from surgery.

> " Eden had her PDA surgery and everything went very well. It took only 15 minutes for the actual procedure and she is recovering nicely. We got to see her post-surgery and she looks peaceful. It was a little scary for me to see her so still from the sedation that she was given. I guess it's better to see her like that than to see her in pain. "
>
> Billie, mother of **Holland** and **Eden**

Low Blood Pressure (Hypotension)

Blood pressure is controlled by a combination of factors, including the tone of the tiny muscles that surround arteries, how much fluid is inside of your blood vessels, and how hard your heart pumps. Babies have lower blood pressures than older children and adults. A healthy preterm baby has even lower normal blood pressures than a healthy full-term baby. Defining a healthy blood pressure for a preterm baby is difficult and depends on the baby's gestational age, age after birth, and health condition. Although it seems like a very basic question, researchers are still trying to determine what a "normal" blood pressure is for a preterm baby and how low a blood pressure can be before it needs treatment.

In the NICU, blood pressure is measured using a tiny blood pressure cuff attached to an electronic machine. If the NICU team needs continuous monitoring of your baby's blood pressure, they may place an arterial line. An arterial line is a special catheter that is threaded into an artery and then attached to an electronic monitor. In the NICU, arterial lines are frequently placed into an artery in the wrist, ankle, or umbilical cord. If placed in the umbilical cord, the line is called an umbilical arterial catheter. (See Chapter 3.)

Treatment of Low Blood Pressure

If treatment is needed, your baby's team will first try to identify which cause of low blood pressure is most likely.

Treatment Options for Low Blood Pressure in Preterm Babies

- Intravenous fluid or blood, called a *volume bolus,* to fill the blood vessels.
- Intravenous medications that increase tone in the tiny muscles around arteries, increase the strength of heart contractions, and increase the heart rate. These medications are often called *vasopressors* (or *pressors*).
- Intravenous steroids, such as *hydrocortisone.* This may be necessary when a baby's blood pressure remains very low despite receiving additional volume and other medications.

Problems Affecting the Preterm Baby's Intestines

The major organs of the gastrointestinal system are the stomach and intestines. The gastrointestinal system is responsible for processing food, absorbing nutrients, and removing waste by making baby's stool. Preterm babies are at risk of a serious intestinal problem called *necrotizing enterocolitis* (*NEC*).

Necrotizing Enterocolitis (NEC)

Necrotizing enterocolitis is a problem in which the cells lining the inside of the intestines become injured and swollen and may die. Damage to the bowel wall may be small or quite serious. In severe cases, a hole may open in the intestinal wall, causing infection of the abdominal cavity and critical illness that can lead to death.

Risk Factors for NEC

Necrotizing enterocolitis is a disease that primarily affects preterm babies; however, some term babies may also get NEC. The more preterm a newborn is at birth, the greater the risk of developing NEC. In the United States, NEC occurs in 4% to 7% of babies with a birth weight less than 1,500 g (3 lb 5 oz).

The reason that babies develop NEC is not completely understood, but NEC most often occurs after babies have begun feedings. Preterm babies who receive only breast milk have a significantly lower risk of developing NEC.

Diagnosis of NEC

Babies with NEC may show a variety of signs, and the early signs may be very subtle. Other babies will have a sudden change in their belly (*abdomen*) and the signs will progress very quickly.

Early signs include abdominal swelling and difficulty digesting feedings. Babies with NEC may have blood in their stool or enlarged loops of bowel you can see by looking at their abdomen. There may be more general signs of illness, including less activity, more apnea, blotchy (*mottled*) skin, and abnormal body temperature.

The most common test for NEC is an abdominal radiograph. Radiographs can identify bowel swelling and signs of gas in the bowel wall or liver. Bacteria invading the injured bowel wall may produce gas, which appears as little bubbles on the radiograph. This sign is called *pneumatosis intestinalis* and confirms the diagnosis of NEC.

Often, the radiograph shows mild problems but does not definitely diagnose NEC. In this case, the NICU team may plan additional radiographs or an abdominal ultrasound. Caregivers may also obtain samples of blood, urine, and spinal fluid looking for signs of infection.

Treatment of NEC

Treatment depends on the baby's signs of illness. If the NICU team is not sure if the baby has NEC, feedings may be stopped and antibiotics given for 24 to 72 hours while additional tests are performed. When feedings are stopped, the caregivers may say the baby is *NPO*. This is a Latin abbreviation that means no feedings are being given by mouth. If the signs of NEC go away and no evidence of NEC is found, feedings may be restarted and antibiotics stopped. This is often called an *NEC scare.*

If the team thinks NEC is likely, your baby may have feedings stopped and antibiotics continued for a week or longer. A tube will be passed through your baby's nose or mouth and into her stomach (*nasogastric* or *orogastric tube*) to drain fluids and allow the intestines to rest. During this time, your baby will receive nutrition through an IV line.

Babies with NEC can be very ill and require close monitoring. Radiographs may be obtained several times a day to check for rupture of the intestinal wall, which would show *free air* in the belly. Your baby may require oxygen or a ventilator for apnea. Additional fluids and medications may be needed for problems with low blood pressure, and your baby may need blood or platelet transfusions.

Most babies with NEC will improve with medications in 48 to 72 hours. Approximately one-quarter to one-half of babies with NEC will continue to get sicker during the first 24 to 48 hours despite medications and will require surgery.

Possible Complications of NEC

Rupture of the intestinal wall is a serious complication of NEC that requires emergency surgery. Surgeons may place a small tube, called a *peritoneal drain,* in the abdomen to allow fluid and pus to drain out. Other babies may need a bigger surgery to open the belly and remove parts of the sick intestine. After surgery, babies may become very unstable and get sicker. Despite antibiotics and surgery, some babies will not get better and will die.

Your baby may come back from surgery with a temporary *ostomy* in place. An ostomy is a surgical opening on the surface of the baby's abdomen where the bowel has been attached so it can drain and have more time to heal. Stool drains from the ostomy opening into a collecting bag.

Babies with severe NEC may need to have a lot of their intestine removed. The amount of healthy intestine left after surgery may be quite short and unable to absorb enough nutrients and water from the baby's food. This is called *short bowel syndrome* or *short gut*. Babies with short gut require prolonged IV nutrition and may need special formula and nutrient supplements.

Several weeks after NEC heals, the bowel wall that was sick may develop scars that narrow the size of the bowel opening. Narrowing of the bowel is called a *stricture*. Babies with strictures have difficulty tolerating their feedings. Their abdomen may become bloated again and they may pass blood in their stool. These complications may require surgery to remove the scarred and narrow bowel.

Problems Affecting the Preterm Baby's Brain

The brain and nervous system begin developing during the third week of pregnancy, and development continues well beyond the second year of life. The brain uses a significant amount of energy and needs a constant supply of blood, nutrition, and oxygen. Because the brain is so complex and it is still developing at the time of preterm birth, it is at risk of injury from many different causes.

Bleeding in the Brain (Hemorrhage)

New brain cells grow in an area deep within the brain called the *germinal matrix*. The germinal matrix sits next to a fluid-filled area of the brain called the *ventricles*. Blood vessels in this area carry a large amount of blood and are very fragile. During the hours before and after preterm birth, changes in blood flow may cause these vessels to break and bleed. The medical term for bleeding is *hemorrhage*. When bleeding occurs, the blood initially collects in the germinal matrix and may also fill the ventricles. The NICU team may call this a *germinal matrix hemorrhage, intraventricular hemorrhage,* or *IVH.*

Risk Factors for Intraventricular Hemorrhage (IVH)

The greatest risk of bleeding in the brain is on the first day of life, and nearly all bleeding (75%) occurs during the first 3 days of life. If a preterm baby has not had an IVH by the end of the first week of life, it is much less likely to occur.

The risk of IVH is directly related to the degree of prematurity and birth weight. Smaller and more preterm babies have a higher risk of bleeding and of the more severe types of bleeding.

The brain's germinal matrix matures between 32 to 36 weeks' gestation, significantly decreasing the risk of this type of bleeding.

Symptoms of IVH

Frequently, babies with a developing IVH have no signs of trouble. However, if the IVH is large, the baby may have a sudden change in her condition, with low blood pressure, seizures, apnea, bradycardia, and a bulging soft spot on the top of the baby's head (*fontanel*).

Diagnosis of IVH

Hemorrhages are diagnosed using an ultrasound scan of the brain. Many NICUs routinely perform an ultrasound during a very preterm baby's first or second week of life even if there are no signs of hemorrhage. The ultrasound scanner is placed on the baby's scalp, over the soft spot, and sound waves are used to create images of the brain. Ultrasound does not expose the baby to any radiation.

If there is bleeding, it will be assigned a grade from 1 to 4 based on the amount of bleeding, its location, and the presence of enlargement or *dilation* of the ventricles. The smallest and most localized type of bleeding is assigned grade 1. More significant bleeds are assigned a higher number. A grade 4 bleed means there is bleeding into the substance of the brain, separate from the germinal matrix and ventricle. If bleeding is present, its progress and the reabsorption of blood will be monitored with ultrasound scans.

Grading Brain Hemorrhages in Preterm Babies

- **Grade 1** is the smallest amount of bleeding. Blood is only in the germinal matrix.
- **Grade 2** means the bleeding has spread into the nearby ventricle.
- **Grade 3** means the blood has entered the ventricles and is enlarging the ventricle.
- **Grade 4** (also called an *intraparenchymal hemorrhage*) means there is bleeding into the substance of the brain, separate from the germinal matrix and ventricle. Often, babies with this type of bleeding also have a large intraventricular hemorrhage.

Complications of IVHs

Most hemorrhages are mild to moderate (grade 1 to 2), and nearly all of these will resolve with few short-term problems. A small percentage of newborns, fewer than 1 in 10, with mild or moderate hemorrhages may develop a blockage of fluid in their brains that causes swelling of the ventricles. This is called *hydrocephalus* or "water on the brain." Some babies with mild or moderate hemorrhages will go on to develop long-term developmental problems, such as cerebral palsy or learning disabilities.

Severe hemorrhages are more likely to result in short- and long-term problems. More than half of babies with grade 3 or 4 hemorrhages will develop hydrocephalus and long-term developmental problems, such as cerebral palsy, hearing loss, vision loss, and learning disabilities.

Hydrocephalus

Spinal fluid surrounds your baby's brain and spinal cord. *Hydrocephalus* occurs when the flow of spinal fluid is blocked or cannot absorb as it should. Following an IVH, blood in the spinal fluid may block the drainage system or scar the membranes that absorb it. The spinal fluid backs up in the ventricles, causing them to expand and push on the surrounding brain tissue.

Periventricular Leukomalacia

Periventricular leukomalacia (PVL) means abnormal development of the white part of the brain near the ventricles. The white part of the brain carries electrical messages between the brain and spinal cord. Periventricular leukomalacia may be seen by ultrasound scan or magnetic resonance imaging and looks like bright spots or small holes in the brain tissue. Even though the injury that caused PVL may have occurred before or shortly after birth, PVL may not be visible by ultrasound for several weeks after birth. Babies with PVL have a high risk of developing cerebral palsy.

Problems Affecting the Preterm Baby's Eyes

Your baby's eyes begin to develop during the first month of pregnancy, but the development is not complete until after birth.

Retinopathy of Prematurity (ROP)

The *retina* lines the inside of the eye. The retina begins developing around 16 weeks of gestation. It starts at the back of the eye and gradually spreads along the inside of the eyeball. The retina is made of living cells and needs a network of blood vessels to develop along with it. This development continues until near a baby's due date. *Retinopathy of prematurity* (*ROP*) is a disease that occurs when abnormal blood vessels grow and spread throughout the developing retina.

Shortly after preterm birth, the normal growth of the retina and its blood vessels temporarily stops. We do not fully understand why this happens, but one factor is the rapid change in the amount of oxygen in the baby's blood after birth. Fetuses receive much less oxygen than babies need after birth.

After several weeks, the preterm baby's retina and blood vessels begin to grow again, but the blood vessels may not grow normally. There may be rapid, irregular growth of new blood vessels. These abnormal blood vessels are fragile and can leak, scarring the retina and pulling it out of position. If the retina is pulled away from the back of the eye, it is called a *retinal detachment*. Retinal detachment is the main cause of severe visual impairment and blindness in ROP.

Risk Factors for ROP

The risk of ROP increases with decreasing gestational age and birth weight. Retinopathy of prematurity is usually seen in babies less than 30 weeks' gestational age. After that, the retinal vessels have developed enough that they are not at risk. More than half of babies delivered at less than 27 weeks' gestation will develop some ROP.

Higher levels of oxygen in the blood might play some role in the development of ROP. Because of this, the blood oxygen saturation (SpO_2) for all preterm babies receiving oxygen is carefully monitored. The goal is to ensure the baby receives enough oxygen to support her body's needs while limiting excess oxygen that may contribute to ROP. Most NICUs use pulse oximetry to monitor oxygen saturation and have target levels that they hope to maintain as long as the baby is receiving supplemental oxygen. In real life, this can be very difficult to do, as babies often have fluctuating oxygen levels.

Even still, ROP develops in some babies with lower oxygen levels and does not develop in some babies with higher oxygen levels. There have even been cases of ROP in babies who did not receive any additional oxygen. Because the cause of ROP is not fully understood, it is not possible to completely prevent this problem or accurately predict which babies will develop ROP.

Diagnosis of ROP

Babies born at less than 30 weeks' gestation or less than 1,500 g (3 lb 5 oz) usually have their eyes examined by an eye specialist (*ophthalmologist*) when they are approximately 4 to 5 weeks old. Some babies weighing 1,500 to 2,000 g or delivered between 30 and 32 weeks' gestation will be examined if their physician thinks they are at risk. In some institutions, photographs of the retina are taken with a special camera and electronically sent to an ophthalmologist for evaluation.

Before the eye examination, drops will be placed in the baby's eyes to enlarge (*dilate*) the pupils so the retina can be viewed. The ophthalmologist uses a special lens to look into the eyes and evaluate the progress of retinal development. The ophthalmologist may simply say the retina is still immature. This means no ROP was seen; however, the retina and its blood vessels are still developing and are at risk of ROP.

If abnormal blood vessels are seen, the ophthalmologist will describe the ROP according to a standard system. The description includes a number that describes the severity of the condition (stage) and a description of which portion of the retina is involved (zone). The term *PLUS disease* is used if the ophthalmologist sees very aggressive ROP with thick and twisted blood vessels. Retinopathy of prematurity may involve only one eye or both. Depending on the maturity of the retina and presence of ROP, the ophthalmologist will schedule additional follow-up examinations.

> ❝ Bad news is that both girls had their eye exams yesterday and the eye doctor says that they have progressed to zone 2, stage 3 ROP, which requires surgery. That means they will go back on the ventilator and be sedated for the surgery. The prognosis for both girls is good, but it's pretty likely that one or both girls will need to wear glasses, maybe at an earlier age than most kids. ❞
>
> Billie, mother of **Holland** and **Eden**

Treatment of ROP

In mild cases, ROP resolves by itself and leaves no permanent damage. Babies with more severe ROP can develop poor vision or even blindness and may require laser surgery. With this treatment, a laser beam directed into the eye destroys the outer areas of the retina, slowing or reversing the abnormal vessel growth. The baby may lose some vision to the side (*peripheral vision*), but the goal of laser surgery is to prevent retinal detachments and save the baby's ability to see straight ahead. Babies with the most advanced ROP who develop a retinal detachment may need additional surgery.

Problems Affecting the Preterm Baby's Skin

Intact skin is an important barrier. It protects the body from invading bacteria, helps maintain fluid balance by preventing excess water loss, and provides insulation, preventing heat loss. Preterm skin is a less effective barrier and more prone to injury than fully mature skin.

The Preterm Baby's Skin

You may notice that a very preterm baby's skin initially appears shiny, sticky, and gelatinous with visible veins. More mature babies have a dry, flaky layer of skin. After birth, preterm skin matures quickly. You will notice your baby's skin becoming dry and flaky. This is a normal and healthy change. Within a few weeks, a preterm baby's skin is similar to the skin of a term baby.

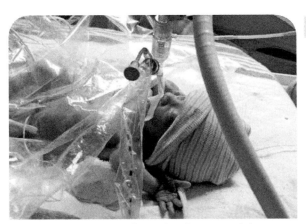

Preterm babies like **Jack**, who are less than 32 weeks' gestation, are covered in plastic wrap or placed inside a polyethylene plastic bag to prevent heat loss at birth.

Heat Loss

At birth, a newborn moves from her mother's warm uterus to the cooler delivery room. For the first time, the newborn must control her own temperature. As far back as the early 1900s, researchers found that carefully maintaining a normal body temperature improved survival of preterm newborns. If preterm newborns use energy for heat production, they may use up their energy stores, develop low blood sugar, and stop growing.

Maintaining a normal body temperature is a major focus of care from the moment of birth. In the delivery room, your baby will be placed under a radiant warmer. Right after birth, babies less than about 32 weeks' gestation may be covered up to their neck with a clear plastic sheet or bag similar to the plastic wrap you use in your kitchen. Shortly after birth, preterm newborns may be moved to an incubator. The incubator keeps your baby warm by controlling the environmental temperature and blocking cool air currents that could move across her body. Very preterm newborns may also have humidity added to the air in the incubator to prevent water loss from the baby's skin.

Special Care for Preterm Skin

All preterm babies receive special skin care. Skin care includes gentle handling; avoidance of lotions, ointments, or other substances (unless medically indicated); use of special tape that is gentle to the skin; avoidance of adhesives; and use of special transparent wound dressings. These clear adhesive dressings can be used over skin irritations to promote healing or over places where IV lines or catheters have been inserted to protect these sites and reduce the risk of infection. A soft, easy-to-remove barrier may be placed between the tape and the newborn's skin.

Even with careful attention to skin care, some preterm newborns may develop areas of skin irritation. Preventing irritation and skin breakdown is an important but challenging goal for neonatal care providers. New research is constantly changing neonatal skin care practices, and each NICU may have its own skin care protocol.

Knowledge Is Power

This chapter has described many common problems that can occur in preterm babies. The wide range of potential problems may seem overwhelming. It is important to remember that being at risk for a problem does not mean a baby will certainly develop it. Many preterm babies will experience one of the problems described in this chapter; some will experience several; and, unfortunately, a few will experience many. Knowledge of your baby's risks for specific problems enables you and your NICU team to monitor your baby carefully, identify signs of developing problems, and begin treatment quickly. Your team can provide more specific information about your baby's risks based on her gestational age, birth weight, and unique health conditions.

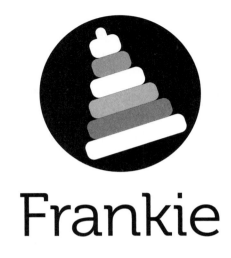

Frankie

Born at 29 weeks

I was admitted to the hospital after a prenatal appointment at 27 weeks' gestation. We actually were told at that appointment that I might be delivering Frankie that evening and from the moment we heard that, we were pretty terrified. I was put on bed rest, diagnosed with preeclampsia. Frankie was delivered via emergency C-section 2 weeks later.

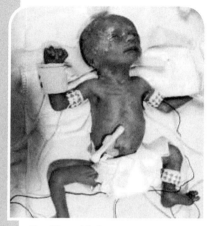

Frankie, at birth.

We knew it would be an emergency C-section. The labor and delivery staff made sure that I understood what that was going to look like. They prepared me with everything I needed to know. It was quick and I was able to see Frankie minutes later. They wheeled my bed in to see her as the nurses and doctors were evaluating and connecting Frankie to all her monitors. Frankie was 1 pound 11 ounces, 14¼ inches long.

I honestly believe I was in complete shock. Everything they told me, I never processed. I know this because my husband recorded many of our conversations with staff, and I don't remember any of it.

Physical exhaustion, mental exhaustion, intravenous magnesium, and now your child is born and you need to produce milk and pump every 3 hours…it's incredibly exhausting. So, ironically, Frankie entered the world during the opening ceremony of the summer Olympics and we were having our own opening ceremony, life of preemie parents in the NICU.

Frankie now weighs 24 pounds and is 3 feet tall. She was born and still is a thriver! While I teach, she learns at an in-home day care 5 days a week. I would have never thought she would be in a day care with GERMS! She counts to 50, spells her name, rides a bike with training wheels, takes ballet, can brush her own teeth, is potty-trained (wow, that was so easy compared to other things), uses technology quite well, loves books, loves the outdoors, and, yes, throws little tantrums!

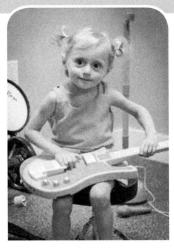

Frankie, at age 3.

It's awesome to see her growth and development with eating and sleeping. Those things were our concern and she has made such fantastic progress. I would have never imagined her cutting her own food, enjoying so many different types of food, but most importantly, she eats with no pain or aversions.

I rarely refer to her as a preemie. She was born a preemie, but she is all toddler now. She is 3½ years old! I will never forget our time spent in the hospital and the challenges we faced for several years. These babies thrive. They can thrive and they do thrive.

Lisa, mother of Frankie

CHAPTER 6

Parenting in the NICU

> "Watching my son fight for his life in the hospital every day was incredibly hard, but the many magical moments I experienced with him as he got healthier and stronger kept me going. I will never forget the first time I held him in kangaroo care while he was still on a ventilator, the first time he took a full feed from a bottle with the breast milk I had pumped, and the first time I gave him a bath in a little bucket."
>
> *Cheryl, mother of **Nathan***

You are an important part of your baby's life in the neonatal intensive care unit (NICU) and a valuable member of your baby's health care team. At first, you may feel nervous around the equipment and NICU staff, but you have a bond with your baby that no other member of the NICU team can match. You will learn how to care for your baby in a context of love that will continue long after the NICU stay is behind you.

There can be many challenges of parenting in the NICU, but you can meet them. A positive experience depends on forming a working partnership with the NICU team and getting involved in your baby's care. This helps you learn about your baby, grow as a parent, and prepare for your baby's homecoming.

Forming a Partnership With the NICU Team

Getting to know the daily NICU routine and providing care for your baby helps break down some of the challenges to NICU parenting. Open and honest communication with the health care team creates trusting partnerships. You are an essential member of your baby's team and your input and involvement are important in planning and carrying out your baby's plan of care. In a successful partnership, planning for your baby's discharge begins early in the NICU stay.

Ask Questions and Learn as You Go

No question is silly or unnecessary. Take as much time as you need to discuss your concerns and questions. Don't be afraid to say that you just don't understand something or need the information presented in a different way. People learn in many different ways and at different paces. The NICU team expects you to have plenty of questions.

Forgetting what you've been told is normal when you're distracted by the NICU environment. Don't be embarrassed or afraid to ask for the information again.

Write Down Questions as You Think of Them

Families often have many questions about their baby, but when they get the chance to ask, no one can remember the questions. To avoid this problem, write down your questions as they occur to you. Keep your list in your purse or wallet, make a reminder on your phone, or start a folder on your tablet so you'll have your questions ready when you need them. You can use the same system to write down the answers to your questions and file them for future reference.

Communication Starters

Starting your questions or ideas with conversation openers can help you reach your goals. These openers allow you to give and receive information at the same time.

- "Would you think about…?"
- "Can you share with me the pros and cons of…?"
- "What if we tried…?"
- "I read about…. Do you think that might work?"
- "I'm not familiar with…. Can you tell me more?"

Questions That Don't Have a Clear Answer

It is important to feel comfortable and satisfied with the answers to your questions. Keep in mind, however, that you may not always get the answer you want. Some questions have no clear answers. In other cases, too many variables exist to permit a specific answer. Lack of a conclusive answer can be frustrating. Acknowledging your frustration to your baby's team may be helpful. Chances are team members are also frustrated when they cannot give a conclusive answer.

> " I am a transgender man and I gave birth to my baby. This NICU respected that I am Pascal's dad, not his mom. For trans or LGB parents who land in the NICU, ask for your pronouns and title to be respected. Post a note for staff near your baby so you don't have to explain over and over. Not worrying about how I would be referred to meant I could focus on him, instead of building a protective wall around that part of my being. "
>
> Alex, father of **Pascal**

Challenges of NICU Parenting

Learning how to touch and hold your baby and read her cues is an important part of parenting. However, NICU parents may feel that obstacles stand between them and their baby. Parenting will get more comfortable as you learn more about your baby and as your baby starts to mature and feel better. In the meantime, it helps to know about common parenting barriers and how to deal with them.

Separation

If your baby is in a NICU some distance from your home, family members may be separated from one another. It may be difficult to find an affordable place to stay near your baby. Low-cost temporary housing is sometimes available for parents. Some hospitals may make rooms available or have arrangements with nearby hotels for parents and family. Ask about these resources and use them when you are able.

If you are parenting from a long distance, set up a phone call schedule and communicate often with your baby's health care team. Strategies to help you cope with long-distance parenting may include joining rounds by phone, using online video systems, or e-mails and photos sent to you to update you on your baby's progress and involve you in your baby's life. Try not to feel guilty if you are not able to be there as much as you would like. Keep in touch with your baby's NICU team—they know you care. For parents at a distance, the chance to room-in (see Chapter 8) before discharge is very valuable. Ask the team about the possibilities.

Exhaustion

Many parents find the overall atmosphere of the NICU stressful and exhausting. Rest is essential for both parents, but for mothers, it's especially important for recovering after childbirth and for milk production. Many NICUs have a parent lounge where parents can go when they are tired or overwhelmed. Your NICU team will tell you where you can rest, recharge digital devices, eat, and use the bathroom.

Devices and Equipment

Many mechanical barriers come between you and your baby in the NICU. Your baby's incubator can be intimidating at first. You may hesitate to break through this barrier and touch your baby. Tubing and monitor wires can tangle like vines in the jungle, and you don't want to risk pulling something loose. All of this can make caring for your baby a challenge, but the NICU team can help you work around these obstacles.

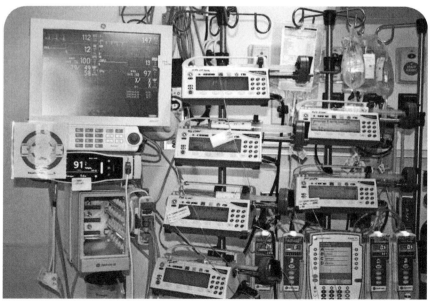

Bedside equipment, such as this wall of pumps and monitors, can be an intimidating obstacle for parents in the NICU.

Psychological Barriers

Parents report a range of emotions about the NICU environment. How you feel may depend on whether you were expecting your baby to need NICU care, your baby's condition, your own condition, and if you have any past NICU experience. When coming into the NICU, it may seem like a foreign land. You may feel uncertain and wonder about any unspoken "rules" or expectations. You may fear that if you ask too many questions or become demanding, you will annoy the staff, and your baby may not receive good care. These fears are normal but unfounded. They will lessen as you become more familiar and involved with the staff and the NICU routine. If your birth didn't happen as you planned, you and your partner may also mourn the loss of that planned birth experience. You may have written a detailed birth plan about how you wanted your labor and delivery to unfold. Unfortunately, your preterm or complicated birth may not have met many of these expectations. Developing a new set of goals for making progress is an important part of NICU parenthood. These new goals may include weaning off of oxygen or breastfeeding for the first time.

> " I came into the NICU with a certain (small!) amount of antagonism. I respected the hospital and medicine in general, but I also had these small voices of doubt and suspicion—did he really need to be there? Were they overreacting? Were they just trying to keep us apart? That made it harder to accept his needs and appreciate the care he was getting at first. "
>
> Alex, father of **Pascal**

Guilt and Anger

For nearly all parents, the NICU is a new and stressful place. Many parents feel guilty after the birth of a baby who needs care in a NICU. You may ask yourself and the NICU team, "What did I do to cause this?" or "What could I have done to prevent this?" Parents examine their lives since the day they learned about the pregnancy, wondering if they could have changed the outcome.

You may feel powerless and angry that your birth experience did not go as expected. You might find yourself angry at your family and friends or even your partner ("They just don't understand."). As uncomfortable as it may be, you may also feel angry at your baby ("Why couldn't you have waited for just a few more weeks?").

It helps to know that most pregnancy and birth complications are not anyone's fault and many NICU admissions are unexpected. Still, many parents feel they may somehow have done something—or not done something—to make it happen. Share these feelings with your NICU team. Often, the NICU team can provide answers and reassurance.

Attachment

Some parents admit feeling jealous of nurses who do everything well and seem to meet their baby's needs better than they can. But as you spend time with your new baby, you will find yourself becoming the expert about her needs. Actively participating in her care will help you feel more like a parent and resolve many of those feelings.

If your baby was very ill, you may also have a lingering fear that your baby could die. This may complicate feelings of love and attachment. Give yourself some time to sort out your feelings, and remember that loving feelings for your baby will grow stronger over time. You may find it helpful to discuss your feelings with your baby's nurse, social worker, or another support person.

> 66 Another thing I have forgiven myself for, but didn't at the time, was my inability to love my son in the first few weeks. At 24 weeks' gestation, he didn't look like the babies you see in pictures or on social media. It was a defense mechanism, I think. I didn't have anyone in my social network who had delivered a baby so early, or even preterm at all. That was isolating. 99
>
> Robyn, mother of **Auggie**

The "Baby Blues" and Postpartum Depression

Pregnancy and childbirth bring about tremendous physical and emotional change, with dramatic variation in maternal hormone levels. These changes may affect brain function and can lead to depression. This is more common than many people realize, and many new mothers experience the "baby blues" to some extent. Symptoms may begin in the early days after the baby's birth and include feeling anxious or irritable, with mood swings. Many mothers find themselves suddenly tearful, and there may be unwelcome changes in appetite or sleep patterns. The "baby blues" should subside within 2 weeks, but sometimes symptoms will come later or extend beyond that time frame. These feelings usually go away on their own and usually do not last for more than 2 weeks.

Postpartum depression is a more serious concern and can occur anytime during the first year after childbirth. It is more common in mothers who experience additional stresses, such as those of parenting a baby with special care needs. Adoptive mothers who have not actually birthed their babies may also find themselves struggling with this common condition. The mother who is experiencing this may not recognize her symptoms or seek help without assistance from her partner or other support person. Your new baby needs parents to be at their best, so it is vitally important to seek expert help if symptoms last longer than 2 weeks. Postpartum depression can occur in men too; research is now showing that up to 10% of dads can experience significant depression in the first year of their baby's life.

Persistent symptoms that signal the need for professional intervention include feeling depressed and disinterested in activities that are usually enjoyable, having a hard time concentrating, and continued feelings of anxiety, guilt, unworthiness, or hopelessness. Some mothers may become so troubled that they consider harming themselves or others. Whether symptoms are mild or severe, postpartum depression can be successfully managed. Talk to your obstetrician, family physician or practitioner, or a member of your NICU team about obtaining professional assistance.

> " I wish I had known earlier that post-traumatic stress disorder (PTSD) is something that NICU parents can experience. I had horrible flashbacks of the events around his birth. "
>
> Robyn, mother of **Auggie**

Your Partner, Your Family, Your Friends

Family Imbalance

This can be a highly stressful time for parents, marked by feelings of physical and emotional separation. Some couples offer each other remarkable support, growing closer and building their bond through this experience. Others may feel separated by anger, guilt, denial, blame, or feelings of failure and uncertainty. Mothers, fathers or partners, and other family members may be doing everything they can to cope with the situation and not have any energy left over to support each other. Many parents say they don't tell each other what they are thinking or feeling. In these cases, stress and misunderstandings can multiply because everyone is too exhausted to sort things out. When issues are not discussed, marriages, partnerships, and family relationships can suffer.

Partners May Cope Differently

After discharge from the hospital, a NICU mother may get less sleep than she needs and be catching meals on the run. Some mothers feel they have more jobs than their partner—and no time for themselves or the rest of the family. The NICU mom may be making daily trips to the NICU and wonder why her partner does not seem more involved.

Some fathers cope by backing off, leaving the mother to assume most of the parenting role. Many men busy themselves at work to restore normalcy and control to their lives. Fathers and others who feel uncomfortable in the NICU may cope with their helplessness by avoiding the NICU.

If parents are feeling stressed but coping in very different ways, it is no wonder their relationship becomes strained. When you are in crisis, you may not have the energy to help others. It can be difficult to talk to one another and understand the other's point of view.

Although open, expressive communication may be difficult, it is important to maintain your relationships. Seek help from other parents who have experienced the NICU, from your spiritual counselor, or from caring professionals. Many couples find they need emotional support and professional assistance to work through difficulties and keep their relationships strong.

It may be hard to take time out for yourself, as well as ask for help; however, taking time is important to restore the energy you need to deal with the NICU. As soon as you feel you are able, take a day off from the NICU, make a date with your partner, and meet your own personal needs. This time-out is essential for your well-being. Don't think of it as taking time away from your baby.

Drugs and alcohol may temporarily help you forget your problems, but they only complicate things in the long run. If you have a substance dependence disorder, you will not likely be able to face the realities of parenting without professional help. If your problems seem overwhelming, seek help from your family health care professional or ask your baby's social worker for help.

> **It's easy to forget to take care of yourself, but if you don't eat and you don't sleep, you can't take care of your kiddo.**
>
> Matthew, father of **Lucy**

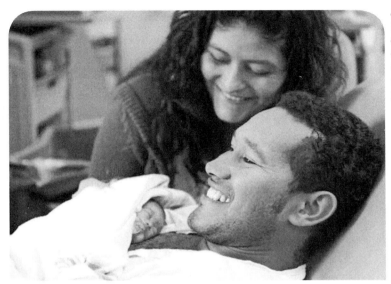

Getting acquainted with your baby takes time. This father is now comfortable enough with the NICU environment to enjoy skin-to-skin care with his baby.

Courtesy of University of Washington Medical Center, Seattle, WA.

What to Tell Your Other Children

If you have other children, they will want to know when the baby is coming home or where the baby is. Tell them as simply as you can about their sibling. Be honest, and try to answer your children's questions at their level. Remember that for younger children, a baby they cannot see is difficult to imagine. Showing them pictures of the baby can help them see her as a real person.

It can be especially difficult for toddlers and preschoolers to understand what is happening. Young children may not understand why their routines are disrupted after the new baby's arrival and say things like, "I hate that baby." These feelings are normal. They also need to be reassured that the baby's illness is not their fault. Simple explanations and "exchanging" gifts with the baby help small children feel important and involved. Some NICUs have sibling support classes, and attending class with you can help toddlers and young children.

You will be understandably upset by the birth of a baby who needs intensive care, and even young children will know something is wrong. If you leave your children out of this experience or neglect to discuss everyone's feelings, they are likely to respond with temper tantrums, crying episodes, or clinging behaviors. Reassure them you will still be able to care for them, and keep them safe and well, despite the current situation. They are likely to manage better if you keep them informed with simple information.

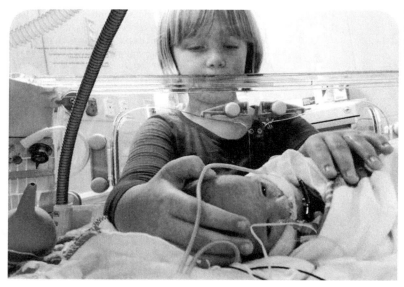

Lydia feels more involved after spending some time with **Bailey Jo** and **Abraham** in the NICU.

Talk to your NICU team about the policies for sibling visitation. Brothers and sisters benefit from visiting the NICU. Rarely are they overwhelmed by the sights and sounds that bother adults. They tend to focus on the little human being who they, too, have been expecting. Actually seeing the baby and the place that is the NICU, along with updates about your baby's progress, will help make the baby real and make siblings feel involved.

Involving Grandparents

You may have wonderful, supportive relationships with both sets of grandparents who step up to the task and help you through the NICU experience with barely any coaching from you. Other NICU parents do not have such great relationships with their own parents and should think carefully about their own needs before inviting their parents to actively participate. If relationships are strained even before the baby comes along, the pressure of NICU care may add layers of stress. Some grandparents think they are being helpful by "taking charge" and doing things that are not helpful to the baby's parents. These grandparents may be surprised at first, but telling them what you really want them to do will pay off. Part of successful family management is knowing when to ask family members for help and support and when to ask them to back off.

Friends

Friends can be a source of stress as well as support. If they fear saying the wrong thing, they may cope by avoiding you and the NICU experience at a time when their support would be helpful. Pregnant friends may feel guilty for being pregnant or having a healthy baby. Just when you need their support, they seem to pull away. This avoidance reflects your friends' feelings of inadequacy, rather than lack of caring. If you feel awkward or do not have the energy to do so, a steadfast friend, your partner, or your parents or partner's parents can tell your friends exactly what you need or how they can help. Friends usually have to be told only once, and then they'll make dinner, pick up your children at child care, run errands, or help in other directed ways.

> In the beginning, you are in such a daze and everyone wants to come visit. I wish I had said no initially—to give us time to get used to our new normal.
>
> Kate, mother of **Lucy**

Keeping Others Informed

There are many ways to keep family members and friends informed of your progress, of good times and hard ones. Some strategies include assigning a person close to you to check in and distribute the message or information that you choose to share. Some hospitals have services that support development of a Web page or update page just for patients and families; these can be easy to build and are secure, and you invite only those you wish to view them. Ask the staff in your NICU about what is available and what has worked for other families.

Support Groups

Sources of support include extended family members, friends, nurses, social workers, the NICU staff, and other NICU parents. You may find that as your needs change over time, so do your support people.

At some point in your NICU stay, you may have questions that can only be answered by someone who has been through the experience. These questions can often be addressed in support groups that are offered at the hospital or in your community. Ask the NICU team if there is a parent-to-parent program or support group available in your community.

Understanding Your Baby

As your baby grows and continues to get stronger, her personality will begin to show. You may be concerned about her ability to use her 5 senses. What are her capabilities? How can you understand what your baby is telling you? Every baby is different, and her gestational age and health problems may influence the answers. The following descriptions apply to many babies in the NICU.

Vision

If a baby is born before 25 weeks of gestation, her eyes may be fused closed at the time of birth. If your baby is born with closed eyelids, no special treatment is necessary. Her eyes will open on their own, on average, within about one week of birth.

There is something very real and magical about looking into your baby's eyes. Parents in the NICU are often overheard saying, "Open your eyes, so I can see you and say hello." Looking into your baby's eyes can be a really special way to connect with your baby.

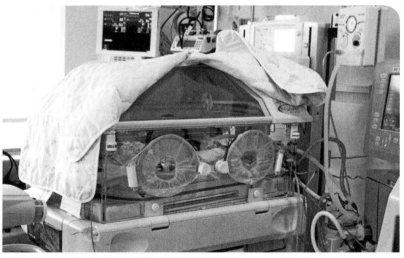

A blanket over the incubator helps block bright light so your baby can rest.

Position your baby face-to-face about 6 to 10 inches away. This is where your baby can see the best, and faces are a baby's favorite thing to look at. Initially, your baby may not be able to look at you and follow your face, but as she grows and remains awake for longer periods, her skills will improve.

> ❝ We had a nice surprise today while visiting Eden. She chose the perfect time to open up both of her eyes and look up at us. We talked to her and we like to think that she looked right at us. We told her what a good girl she is and how pretty she looks with her eyes open. It was a really awesome moment for both of us. ❞
>
> Billie, mother of **Holland** and **Eden**

Hearing

The ears begin to develop in the fourth week of gestation, and the sense of hearing continues to develop until the baby reaches term. As your baby grew during pregnancy, she was exposed to a variety of sounds, such as your heartbeat. Your baby can recognize your voice and, as she gains strength, she may turn toward you when you speak. Some parents find it helpful to provide audio recordings with soothing sounds, including soft music or themselves reading or talking. Many NICU staff find that parents' voice recordings help the baby to quiet and settle down to sleep.

Smell and Taste

Your baby has a well-developed sense of smell and taste. When feeding, she may prefer the taste of her mother's milk and recognize her parents' unique odor. Some units give mothers (and sometimes their partners too) small cloth pads to wear and then place them in bed with their baby. This may comfort the baby and helps the baby recognize the mother's smell in anticipation of breastfeeding.

Touch

The sense of touch develops very early before birth. Your baby is able to feel cloth against her skin and the warmth of your skin against hers. Your baby's face, the area around the lips, and the hands are especially sensitive to your touch. Touching your baby is a wonderful way to connect and help care for your baby. You can help quiet your baby with a firm touch or by holding her hand. Sometimes, babies are annoyed by stroking with your fingertips, perhaps because it feels like a tickle. Watch your baby as you touch her and see what kind of touch helps her relax.

In addition to touching your baby, you can give her a sense of security by providing boundaries. Inside the uterus, your baby was surrounded and contained by the uterine wall. You can comfort your baby in that same way by placing your warm hands against her feet and on top of her head or by gently holding her hands across her chest. Your baby's nurse can show you different ways to "contain" your baby, and you will learn what your baby likes best.

Babies also like a "nest," made of soft surfaces, as they lie in bed. Some units use special buntings or sleeping bags to provide *containment,* or your NICU nurses may place soft rolled blankets around your baby. Your baby will not need these soft quilts and nesting materials by the time she's ready to go home. Unless your baby has medical needs for a special sleep position, your baby will sleep on her back on a firm mattress without any extra bedding or blankets before discharge, and this will continue at home.

Your baby can feel pain, and pain control is an important part of NICU care. Nurses know to watch for signs of discomfort, such as facial expressions and increased heart rate, respiratory rate, blood pressure, and oxygen use. Ask your NICU team what strategies are being used to help keep your baby comfortable, as well as what you can do to help.

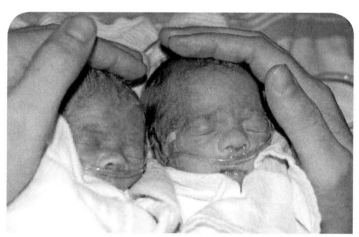

Lukas and **Gabbie** calm with their dad's firm touch.

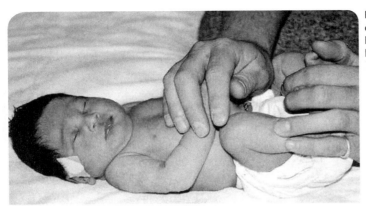

Babies appreciate boundaries. This father can calm his baby by gently holding the baby's arms and legs securely against his body.

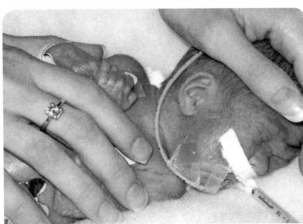

Holland's mother provides secure boundaries by touching Holland's head and snuggling Holland's arms to her chest.

Nathan feels secure in his "nest."

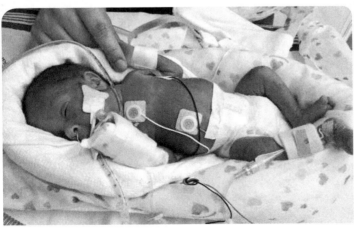

Your Baby's Personality

As you spend more time with your baby, you will become aware of her unique personality and methods for communicating likes and dislikes. To understand your baby's behavior, it is helpful to understand infant behavioral states and cues.

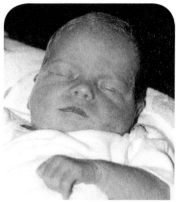

Deep sleep. The baby is very difficult to awaken from deep sleep.

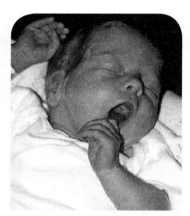

Light sleep. The baby may move around, even fuss a little, in this state, but she is not fully awake.

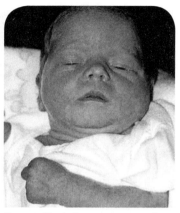

Drowsy. The baby may open and close her eyes and move her arms and legs. By holding her upright and talking to her, you may be able to alert her. If left alone, she may go back to sleep.

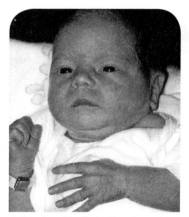

Quiet alert. The baby "brightens" and focuses on your face or voice. As your preterm baby matures, her quiet alert periods will increase.

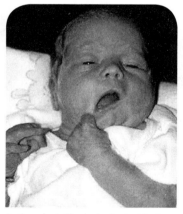

Active alert. The baby is alert but may become fussy and overwhelmed. If you decrease stimulation, she may recover and return to a quiet alert state.

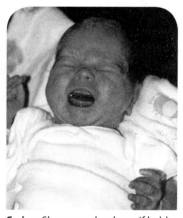

Crying. She may calm down if held securely in quiet surroundings, given a pacifier or her fingers to suck on, or fed if she is hungry.

Behavioral States

Newborns experience 6 different levels of awareness called *behavioral states*. Your baby's state influences how she responds to people and the environment. An ill or preterm baby will show the same behavioral states as a healthy term baby, but these states may not be as easily recognized and transition from state to state may not be as smooth.

Deep Sleep

In deep sleep, your baby breathes regularly. Her eyes are closed, with no noticeable eye movements. She does not move much but may startle or jerk. Your baby is difficult to arouse, unable to respond to most stimulation, and not interested in eating.

Light Sleep

In light sleep, also known as *rapid eye movement* or *REM sleep,* your baby may breathe irregularly. Her eyes remain closed, but eye movements can be seen beneath the lids. Some activities, such as sucking movements, are common in light sleep. Your baby may fuss during this state and can be awakened enough to feed. This state is seen more clearly beginning at 36 weeks' gestation.

Drowsy

In the drowsy state, your baby may open her eyes, or her eyelids may flutter. She may move her arms and legs, and her breathing may become rapid and shallow. If you speak to her or hold her upright, your baby may move from drowsiness into the quiet alert state. If you leave her alone, she may go back to sleep.

Quiet Alert

In the quiet alert state, your baby has a "bright" look and is able to focus her attention. This is the ideal state for interacting with your baby. Preterm babies can reach the quiet alert state but, often, only for seconds. As your baby matures, her periods of quiet alertness will increase.

Active Alert

Your baby's activity increases in this state. Reacting to sound, touch, or movement, she may startle and thrust her arms and legs. Her breathing can be irregular, and she may be fussy. She is unable to focus attention for very long. If you continue to speak to your baby or try to make eye contact, she may start to cry. If you offer rest and containment, she may return to the quiet alert state.

Crying

Crying tells you that your baby has exhausted her coping skills. Your baby needs to rest or needs relief from pain, discomfort, or hunger.

Behavioral Cues

When you learn to recognize your baby's state, you will begin to recognize the best times to interact or play with her.

Invitation Cues

These cues say, "I'm ready." Your baby usually shows invitation cues when in the quiet alert state.

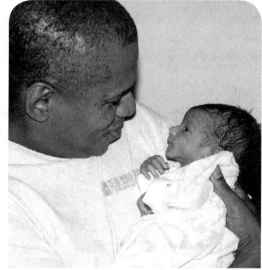

Baby Invitation Cues

- Bright look
- Relaxing hands, arms, legs
- Bringing hands to mouth
- Sucking on fingers, fist, or pacifier
- Making an "ooh" face by pursing lips
- Smiling or cooing
- Looking eye-to-eye, listening, watching your face

This baby is in a quiet alert state. He encourages his father to continue the interaction with invitation cues, such as his bright expression, good eye contact, and relaxed hand position.

Stress Cues

Not only will babies tell you when they are ready to interact, but they will tell you when they have had enough or are not in the mood. Babies show stress cues when they become tired or uncomfortable. Sometimes, your baby simply needs a short break, while other times, your baby is telling you she is ready to sleep or to be left alone.

As you interact with your baby, you may begin to notice some of these stress cues. Your baby may be telling you it's time to stop socializing for now.

Baby Stress Cues

- Startling, jerking, or twitching
- Coughing, sneezing, yawning, or sighing
- Hiccupping, gagging, or grunting
- Squirming, turning away, arching
- Frantic or disorganized activity

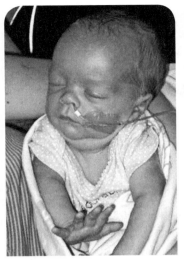

This baby is signaling a need for a break by closing her eyes, turning her head away, and splaying her fingers.

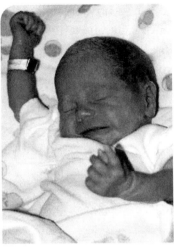

This baby's closed eyes, frowning face, stiff arms, and squirming body are clear stress signals. If swaddled and given total quiet, she may recover a quieter state.

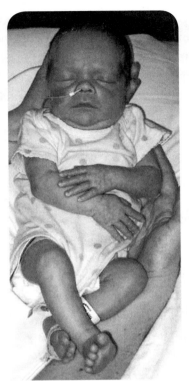

This same baby shows increasing skill at self-comforting by flexing her arms to her midline and bracing her feet.

Mixed Messages

Your baby may demonstrate a mixture of cues. For example, your baby may appear to be in the quiet alert state, ready to interact, yet at the same time be hiccupping. This mixture of cues can be frustrating and confusing. Do you act on the invitation to interact, or do you stop what you are doing and give your baby a break?

If your baby is sending out mixed messages, look for other cues to help you decide whether to interact. For example, if your baby has sent out several invitation cues but then spits up, she may have just finished eating and needed to burp. Now that she has burped (which caused the spit-up), she is again ready for interaction. If, on the other hand, she burps and begins to look tired and turns her gaze away from you, it's probably time for rest. With practice and experience, you'll learn what your baby is telling you in different situations.

As you spend more time with your baby, she will recognize you with all her senses: touch, sound, smell, sight, and taste. At the same time, you will start to recognize what your baby likes and dislikes. Talk with your NICU team about the cues you see and what you have learned about your baby. For instance, you may notice that your baby sleeps better on her right side or spits up less when held upright after feeding. These "little" things are subtle but just as important to your baby's care as things the staff may note about the baby.

Connecting With Your Baby

Babies and children learn through interacting with others. In the beginning, this interaction may be considered "playing" with your baby, and play is often seen as easy, natural, and requiring

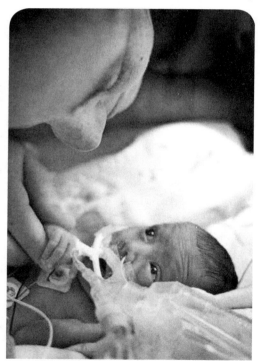

This baby connects with her mother by making eye contact and grasping her finger. Most preterm newborns can sustain this interaction only briefly, but these moments are enriching for the baby and rewarding for her mother.

Courtesy of Gigi O'Dea.

little thought. However, learning to play with your preterm or hospitalized baby may take some time. Initially, you may feel awkward, but as you become more familiar with your baby and see positive responses, you will look forward to your time together.

One Thing at a Time

Follow your baby's lead. If your baby is showing invitation cues, let her look at your face or hear your voice. *Introduce only one thing at a time.* Speaking into a baby's face is instinctive for most of us, but it makes the baby look *and* listen. Speak to your baby first, and then watch for the reaction. When your baby hears your voice, her eyes may brighten and she may turn her head to find you. At that point, she is ready to see your face. If your baby is very preterm or ill, she may not tolerate seeing a face and hearing a voice or hearing your voice and being touched at the same time. She may quickly show signs of stress. As she stabilizes medically and grows, she will gradually learn to handle more interaction.

Nonnutritive Sucking

Another important learning activity for your baby is nonnutritive sucking. This type of sucking does not provide nutrition; rather, your baby sucks on her finger or thumb, a pacifier, or your own clean finger, or at a breast after pumping. Nonnutritive sucking helps your baby comfort herself and "organize" her behavioral states, gain weight, improve her feeding skills, and decrease her oxygen needs.

Positioning

Positioning may be used to help your baby stay calm, focused, and "organized" in her behavioral states. Term newborns prefer to curl up in a flexed position, but preterm newborns may not be able to flex their limbs and keep them flexed without assistance. Flexing your baby forward and bringing her arms and legs to the center of her body can help her discover comfort behaviors, such as finger or hand sucking. Body containment, by swaddling and nesting, helps your baby feel safe and secure and promotes normal growth and development. Your NICU team will teach you how to hold and position your baby properly.

Skin-to-Skin Care (Kangaroo Care)

Ask your baby's NICU team when you can hold your baby skin-to-skin, which is called *kangaroo care* in some NICUs. Kangaroo care was developed in South America as a way to keep preterm newborns warm. Mothers were instructed to hold their diapered preterm newborns skin-to-skin beneath their clothing for warmth and breastfeeding. While many NICUs now call the practice *skin-to-skin care*, the term *kangaroo care* has been affectionately maintained in some units.

Mothers and their partners can experience skin-to-skin care. Most nurseries have comfortable rocking chairs and screens that can be placed around your chair or the baby's care area. Simply wear clothing that opens down the front. You will snuggle your baby upright on your chest or lay your baby with her head against your chest.

The benefits of skin-to-skin care for the newborn include warmth, stability of heartbeat and breathing, increased time spent in the deep sleep and quiet alert states, decreased crying, increased weight gain, and improved breastfeeding. These benefits occur even when skin-to-skin care occurs for only a few minutes each day. At a time when so many people are caring for your baby, skin-to-skin care provides special moments of closeness and comfort that only you can experience with your baby.

Skin-to-Skin (Kangaroo) Care

Skin-to-skin care is a fundamental expression of parenting. It is important for mothers and their partners.

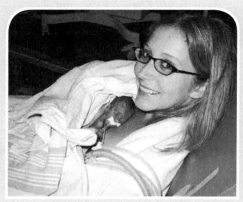

"Today **Eden** took a long nap on Mom during her first kangaroo session. Both of us really enjoyed it!"

*Billie, mother of **Holland** and **Eden***

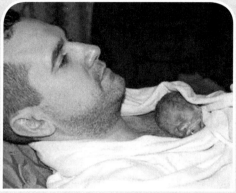

"The most amazing thing about kangaroo care with **Niklas** was watching his vital signs actually improve while laying on my chest!"

*Jason, father of **Niklas, Gabbie,** and **Lukas***

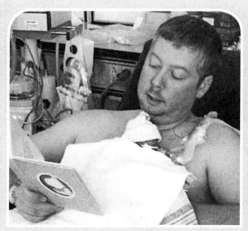

"**Auggie** was always very relaxed and calm during our kangarooing. I looked forward to each opportunity. Here we are reading the *Belly Button Book* by Sandra Boynton. To this day, Auggie likes to start his day by grabbing a book off his shelf and asking me to read it to him."

*Edward, father of **Auggie***

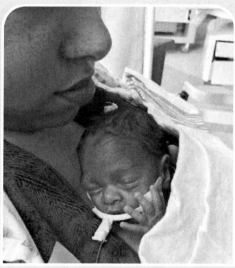

"I will never forget the first time I held him in kangaroo care while he was still on a ventilator…."

*Cheryl, mother of **Nathan***

Growing With Your Baby

During your baby's stay in the NICU, you'll notice how she is growing—physically as well as developmentally. During that time, parents will grow as well. Celebrate accomplishments and "firsts": the first time you hold your baby, the first time you bathe her, the first time you feed her. You may wish to capture these moments in a special baby book of photos and memories that mark progress during your baby's NICU stay. Enjoy the special time you have with your baby. Although this is probably not the way you had imagined becoming acquainted, it can be a memorable and special experience.

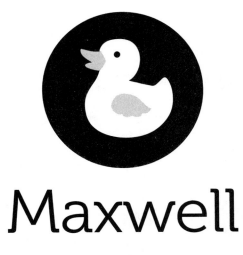

Maxwell

Born at 34 weeks

Our 22-day stay in the NICU was a nerve-racking, challenging time. We went from being at home preparing for baby, to emergency C-section and not knowing if our baby would survive, to living in the hospital with a 5½-pound newborn who was struggling to breathe, suck, and swallow and maintain his body temperature. Looking back now, it was truly amazing to see him develop and grow before our eyes and get stronger each day. We were growing as parents too. We were kind of thrown into the deep end of the pool, paddling to survive.

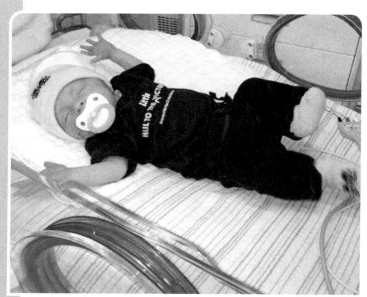

Maxwell in his going-home outfit.

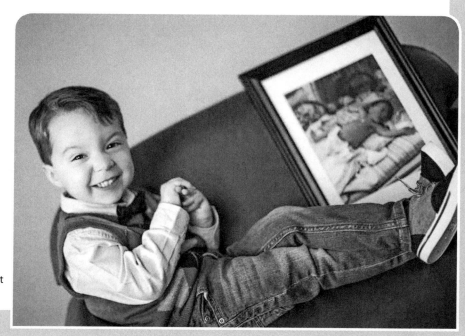

Maxwell, at age 3 years, sitting next to his NICU photo.

The NICU is an amazing place where amazing medicine happens. It can also be an extremely lonely place. Without the empathy and compassion from the doctors and nurses, I'm not sure how anyone could survive those first few weeks.

Maxwell is a healthy 3-year-old today. He still has underdeveloped lungs and gets infections like croup quite often. He also had some delays. He didn't walk until 18 months and he didn't get all of his baby teeth until age 3.

We are so proud of our little man and look forward to all of the great things he will accomplish in his life.

Amanda and Gabriel, parents of Maxwell

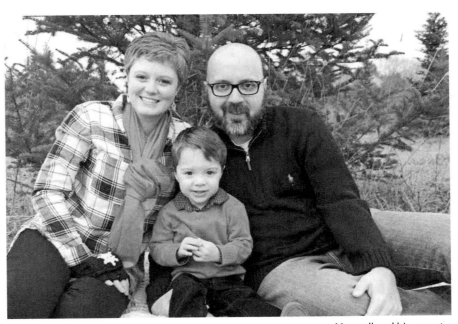

Maxwell and his parents.

CHAPTER 7

Feeding Your Baby

> "Once Sienna no longer needed assistance breathing, it seemed like she was ready to come home! She was bright-eyed and seemed to be looking at me, wondering why she had to stay. This was a difficult phase of the NICU. It was a waiting game, as she learned how to suck, swallow, and breathe at the same time. I got frustrated with the baby steps. Looking back, it was the absolute best thing in the world for her to have stayed there as long as she did."
>
> *Kaitlynn, mother of **Sienna***

Feeding your baby is an important parenting task and a satisfying activity you will want to share with your baby; however, right after birth, your baby may not be able to feed directly from the breast or bottle. Many babies in the neonatal intensive care unit (NICU) will receive nourishment in different ways for some period of time.

Your Baby's First Nutrition

You may be amazed at how hard your tiny newborn can suck on your finger or a pacifier shortly after birth, but it doesn't mean he is ready to begin breastfeeding or bottle-feeding. Criteria for oral feeding vary among units, but, commonly, babies in the NICU will start oral feeding attempts when they are clinically stable, breathing without difficulty, and showing oral feeding cues. Frequently, this occurs when preterm babies are close to 32 to 34 weeks' gestation but may occur earlier. Once babies start oral feeding attempts, it may be a while before they have the skills to suck, swallow, and breathe in a coordinated way. Feeding a sick or preterm baby in the NICU can be a slow and deliberate process with potential complications. Until breastfeeding or bottle-feeding is safe, your baby will be nourished in other ways.

Intravenous Nutrition

Your baby may not be fed by mouth immediately after birth. Instead, he may get his nutrition through an *intravenous* (*IV*) line. If your baby is very preterm or will not be able to begin oral feedings for several days, *total parenteral nutrition* (*TPN*) will likely be used. *Parenteral* refers to nutrition that enters the body through a blood vessel. In TPN, all of the essential nutrients (sugar, protein, fat, vitamins, and minerals) are provided through one of the baby's veins.

Gavage Feeding

Babies are able to suck long before they are able to coordinate the process of sucking, swallowing, and breathing. They get their breast milk (sometimes called *human milk*) or formula through a *gavage tube* or *feeding tube* that is inserted through the nose or mouth and passed down into the stomach. The most common methods of gavage feeding use a tube through the mouth into the stomach (an *orogastric* tube) or use a tube through the nose into the stomach (a *nasogastric* tube). Giving your baby a pacifier to suck on during gavage feeding may help strengthen the muscles used for sucking, cause better weight gain, and reduce the length of hospital stay.

To start, your baby may receive very small amounts. These small feedings are intended to get his stomach and intestines ready to absorb the nutrients in milk. Your baby may receive milk on a regular schedule, such as every 2 or 3 hours (*intermittent* gavage feeding), or may receive milk from a feeding pump that provides a steady flow through the gavage tube (*continuous* feeding). Babies who are gavage fed are carefully watched to make sure they are tolerating the feedings. The baby is watched for bloating (*distention*) of the abdomen and for vomiting.

As your baby becomes ready, he gradually gets larger amounts of milk. As the amount of milk is increased, the amount of IV fluid or TPN is slowly decreased. When your baby is taking all of the milk he needs for growth, he is said to be on *full feedings.* At that point, he no longer needs an IV, except perhaps for medications.

> Eden had another wonderful day today. She is up to 6 mL of breast milk every 3 hours. That's halfway to full feeds! She should start getting fatter any day now. Both babies are at 1 pound 8 ounces. Today is their 4-week birthday. I can't believe so much time has passed. Twenty-eight days with many more to come…and every one of them a blessing.
>
> Billie, mother of **Holland** and **Eden**

Benefits of Breast Milk

Providing breast milk for your sick or preterm baby is perhaps the most important thing you can do for your baby's health. In almost all cases, you'll be able to feed your breast milk to your baby until he is able to nurse. Providing breast milk to a preterm baby can be challenging during the NICU experience, but looking back, parents of babies in the NICU feel the advantages were worth the extra effort.

For most babies in the NICU, breast milk is the best choice. Breast milk provides protection from infections, allergies, and other diseases. If necessary, babies in the NICU can be fed formula that is made from cow's milk or soybeans, but for most NICU babies, formula cannot provide the benefits they receive from breast milk. If maternal milk is not available, your baby may be given donor breast milk (see Can I Use Donated Breast Milk for My Baby? later in this chapter) or formula designed for preterm babies.

Benefits of Breast Milk

- Breast milk produced by women who deliver prematurely differs from that produced after a full-term pregnancy and has more of the nutrients, such as protein, that a preterm baby needs. However, preterm newborns often require additional nutrients, which are given by adding certain nutrients (*fortifying breast milk*).

- Nutrients in breast milk are absorbed more easily than the nutrients made from cow's milk or soybeans.

- Feeding preterm newborns breast milk decreases the risk of a serious intestinal illness (necrotizing enterocolitis) and eye disease (retinopathy of prematurity).

- Neurodevelopmental outcomes of preterm newborns are improved by feeding breast milk.

- Breast milk contains substances that protect a baby from infection.

- Breastfeeding decreases the risk of ear infections, diarrhea, and serious colds.

- Breastfeeding reduces the risk of sudden infant death syndrome (SIDS), allergies and asthma, celiac disease, inflammatory bowel disease, obesity, type 1 diabetes mellitus (also known as juvenile-onset diabetes), and childhood leukemia.

Help Your Baby Get Ready for the Breast or Bottle

You can help your baby develop oral feeding skills by using the following techniques:

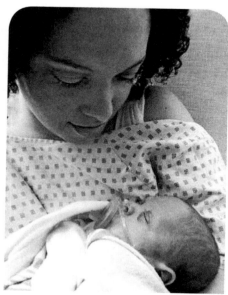

Nonnutritive Sucking

Sucking that does not supply nutrition is called *nonnutritive sucking*. This is good sucking practice and helps weight gain and digestion. Nonnutritive sucking also helps the baby develop self-calming skills.

Watch for signs that your baby would like to suck. These feeding cues include bringing his hands close to his mouth, turning his head and opening his mouth, and making sucking motions. Nonnutritive sucking can occur if your preterm baby nuzzles at your breast during skin-to-skin care (see Chapter 6), but you can slip your clean finger into his mouth on top of his tongue and gently stroke the roof of his mouth with the pad of your finger, or give your baby a pacifier or his fingers to suck anytime he is awake and alert.

Nathan is using a pacifier to practice sucking and develop self-calming skills.

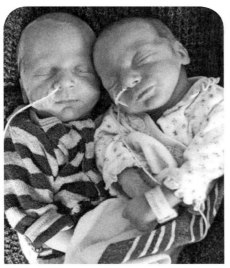

"**Reece** and **Allison** are 15 days old. They are receiving no respiratory assistance, their PICC lines have been removed, and they have overcome jaundice. They are still relying on their feeding tubes."

*Gudrun, mother of **Allison** and **Reece***

Patience and Practice

Depending on your baby's gestational age and health, he may be fed only by gavage tube for several days, weeks, or even months. If you move too quickly to breastfeeding or bottle-feeding, he will get tired, lose weight, and have difficulty staying warm as he uses all his energy to eat. This transition stage from gavage feeding to breastfeeding or bottle-feeding can be frustrating for parents.

When your baby is ready to feed with a nipple, he will try the breast or bottle while the NICU team assesses his skills. Some NICUs have protocols for step-by-step increases in breastfeeding or bottle-feeding. Some feedings will go well; others will be more difficult. The nurses can help you find those times of day when your baby is most awake, alert, and showing signs of readiness to breastfeed.

Learning to eat takes time—it doesn't happen overnight. A growing preterm baby may feed well once but may not again for another day or longer. Many preterm babies can breastfeed fairly well by the time they reach their full-term due date, but many will go home with a combination of breastfeeding and bottle-feeding.

> ❝ I grew more confident as I got to know Lucy and her care team. Sometimes it may feel like you don't have a say in the process, but I learned we were Lucy's voice and needed to speak up even when we didn't know exactly what to say. ❞
>
> Kate, mother of **Lucy**

Providing Breast Milk for Your Baby

Providing breast milk for your baby is one of the most important things you can do for your baby's health. Every family has a lot to think about after labor and birth are over. Amid all the activity, be sure to tell your caregivers that you are planning to breastfeed your baby.

How the Breasts Make Milk

To appreciate the importance of pumping your breasts often and completely, it helps to have an understanding of how breasts work.

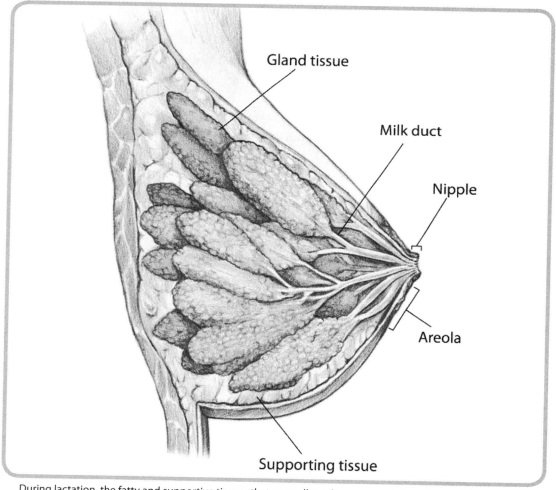

During lactation, the fatty and supportive tissues that normally make up most of the volume of the breast are replaced by glandular tissue necessary to produce milk.

Shortly after a woman gives birth, breasts start producing a thick, clear or yellow-gold liquid called *colostrum*. Within 2 or 3 days after delivery, the colostrum begins to change to a thinner, whiter milk. On about day 3 or 4, maternal hormones cause the breasts to get swollen, hard, and painful. When this happens, people may say that the "milk is coming in." This happens whether the baby is born early or on time and whether the mother breastfeeds or not.

When a baby nurses or when a woman manually *expresses* milk (uses her hands to squeeze it out) or uses a breast pump to suction the milk out, the brain releases 2 hormones. *Prolactin* causes the milk glands in the breasts to start secreting milk, and *oxytocin* causes contractions of tiny muscles that surround the milk glands in the breasts. These contractions squeeze the milk down to the nipples. This is called the *milk-ejection reflex* or the *letdown reflex*. An early sign that this is occurring may be menstrual-like cramps. These cramps are noticeable only in the first week or two after birth, and a mother may not notice them at all if this is her first baby. After a week or so, the mother may notice a feeling of thirst a few minutes after beginning to pump, a tingling sensation or "pins and needles" in the breasts, or milk dripping from the nipples. After pumping, the mother may notice distinct softening of the breasts.

What to Expect in the First Few Days

Soon after a mother gives birth to a baby who is admitted to the NICU, the nurse will provide a breast pump. If the mother's medical condition allows, it is ideal to start within the first 6 hours after giving birth. The nurse will explain how to hold the milk-collecting cups to the breasts and turn on the pump. At first, using the breast pump may feel awkward and embarrassing—and possibly discouraging when only a drop or two of milk appears on the nipple. But every drop is precious, and this first milk is sometimes called "liquid gold." Save every drop in a small container. The volume of your baby's first feeding is very small, perhaps only 1 to 2 mL (about ¼ teaspoon).

In the first few hours after giving birth, especially with everything happening to your baby, trying to learn about pumping and storing milk may feel overwhelming. This is not the best time to take in new information. Don't be ashamed to ask questions and repeat them until you understand the answers. Watch videos if they are available, and ask for written materials to read on your own schedule. Arrange to have your partner, a family member, or a friend in the room when the nurse or lactation consultant is explaining everything; chances are that between you, you'll remember the important points.

> Stick with the pumping for as long as you possibly can. Work with the lactation consultants and your nurses and let them know you want to breastfeed—they are there to help you succeed.
>
> Kate, mother of **Lucy**

Pumping Breast Milk

This is a list of basic information. Your nurses and lactation specialist will provide you with more information.

- Pump both breasts 8 to 10 times a day for about 15 minutes at a time, even if only a drop or two comes out. The milk supply will increase by the third to fifth day. Help to open the ducts and increase milk flow by applying a warm, moist compress and gently massaging the breast before and during pumping.

- Do not let the breasts feel full between pumping, as this can decrease milk supply. If you decide that sleep is more important than pumping, don't let more than 6 hours go by without pumping, and pump at least 8 to 10 times during waking hours. Do not skip pumping at night very often.

- Do not use a small hand-operated or battery-powered pump. Only a hospital-quality, fully automatic electric pump is adequate for the job. Pump both breasts at the same time. This not only saves time but also increases prolactin levels. The hospital will have breast pumps for use while in the NICU. Ask about renting a hospital- grade pump for use at home. Your insurance or Medicaid may help with rental costs.

- Ask your nurse or lactation consultant for advice about storing milk at home and how to bring milk to the NICU. You may pack it in a small cooler, or, for long-distance travel, you may be asked to pack it in dry ice in a sturdy, insulated container.

- Breast milk is not sterile, but it must stay clean. Clean the breast pump parts well, wash hands before pumping, and follow the instructions from your nurse or lactation specialist. If you are unsure about any cleaning or pumping procedures, ask for help.

- The NICU staff may provide printed labels or a bar code to use on the containers. They will check the label or scan the bar code before giving the milk to your baby to reduce the chance of giving your baby another mother's breast milk.

- Your nurses or lactation consultant will teach you how to thaw and warm breast milk in the NICU and after your baby comes home.

- Continue to pump when the baby begins to breastfeed in the NICU. Ask the NICU team when to pump if you know which feeding times your baby will try breastfeeding.

When Not to Breastfeed

Most babies benefit from their mother's milk; however, in some situations, it may not be safe to breastfeed your newborn. Babies with a rare metabolic disease called *galactosemia* should not receive breast milk. Mothers who should not breastfeed include those with HIV. Breastfeeding should not occur if the mother has untreated active tuberculosis (TB) or has active herpes lesions on her breasts; however, expressed milk can be used because there is no concern about these infectious organisms passing through the milk. There are some medications that make breastfeeding unsafe, so you should let your NICU team know about all drugs you are taking. In addition, breastfeeding is not recommended for mothers who use illegal drugs. Mothers can usually breastfeed if they are enrolled in a supervised methadone maintenance program and have negative screening results for HIV and illicit drugs.

Can I Use Donated Breast Milk for My Baby?

The evidence is clear that breast milk is beneficial for the health and development of preterm babies, and many NICUs strive to give preterm and ill babies 100% breast milk. This sometimes requires the use of donated breast milk from a milk bank. The American Academy of Pediatrics recommends using mother's own milk whenever possible, but if a mother's own milk is not available, pasteurized donor milk is the next best choice. The United States and Canada have a growing number of milk banks supervised by the Human Milk Banking Association of North America (HMBANA). Milk banks screen donors to make sure they are healthy and do not have diseases that could be transmitted in their milk. The women who donate to HMBANA milk banks are volunteers who do not get paid for their generous gift. The milk is gently heated and pasteurized to destroy bacteria, while preserving most of the milk's important qualities. The milk is tested for bacterial growth and when it passes its quality testing, it is frozen and shipped to hospitals and individuals who need it. If donor milk is used for your preterm newborn, it should come from a certified milk bank to ensure your baby's health and safety and not from friends, neighbors, or the Internet.

The process for obtaining donor milk varies among hospitals. In many hospitals, a medical order and parental consent are needed to use donor breast milk. At this time, it costs about $4.50 per ounce—more expensive than formula, but this is inexpensive compared to its potential benefits. Some hospitals pay the extra cost for donor milk from a regulated milk bank, but many do not. Your insurance and Medicaid may not cover the cost either. Talk with your NICU team about using donated milk if you cannot provide all the milk your baby needs. It is well worth the effort to give your preterm baby breast milk.

If You Have Had Breast Surgery

Breast implants usually do not interfere with breastfeeding, unless breast damage occurred from the surgery. Breast reduction always affects milk production, but you may be able to produce some milk depending on the type of surgery that was performed. Talk with your baby's lactation specialist about your breast surgery and what you can expect.

Learning to Breastfeed

Learning to breastfeed is a skill for mother and baby. Getting comfortable enough to nurse in the NICU adds a little more stress. Be patient and give yourself a lot of time to learn. Many babies in their early days seem to sleep through the experience. Your patience will pay off. Gradually, your baby will show more interest in nursing and you will gain confidence with your skills.

The best way to learn to breastfeed your baby is to ask the nurse or lactation specialist to help you. They can answer your questions and help with another set of hands and arms until you can manage alone.

Here is a list of basic tips that may be helpful as you and your baby learn what works best for you.

- Sit in a comfortable chair and rest your feet on a small footstool.

- A pillow on your lap may help bring the baby level to your breast. Do not hunch over to nurse a baby in your lap.

- Two common positions for breastfeeding work especially well for preterm babies.

  - **The cross-cradle hold:** Lay your baby on his side facing you, with his mouth right beside your nipple. Encircle your baby's body with the arm opposite the breast that your baby is about to nurse from, and grasp the back of the baby's lower head, neck, and shoulder blades in your hand. With the same-side hand (for example, left hand on left breast), cup your breast by placing your 4 fingers underneath and your thumb on top of your breast.

  - **The football or clutch hold:** Place the baby on a pillow with his legs pointing toward the back of the chair or bed. The same hand as the side of the breast you plan to offer will support the baby's head, neck, and shoulder. The baby is brought up to the breast in a gentle motion toward the nipple. The opposite hand is used to lift and guide the breast for the baby.

- Find a comfortable hand position for holding the breast as you offer the nipple to the baby and support your breast as your baby nurses. Your breast is most likely so heavy that it will pull out of the baby's mouth if you don't support it.

  – With your fingers cupping your breast, press the dark area around the nipple (the *areola*) to fit your baby's mouth. Although the mouth forms a circle when open wide, as soon as it clamps onto your areola and nipple, the lips and gums form a flattened oval. If you gently compress your breast in that same oval shape, your baby is likely to be able to suck longer. Keep your thumb and fingers a little behind the areola so they are not in the way of your baby's mouth. Think about how you squeeze a very thick sandwich just before you take a bite or how you turn an oval peg to fit it into an oval hole. Be sure that your thumb is parallel to your baby's upper lip and your index finger is parallel to your baby's lower lip.

  – Some mothers find a U-shaped hold works better than a C-shaped hold, to ensure the weight of the breast does not interfere with the baby's ability to suckle and for the hand to provide additional jaw support. The U-hold is achieved by placing the thumb on one side of the breast behind the areola, with other fingers placed on the opposite side. In other words, slide your fingers toward the center of your body and your thumb toward the outside of your breast.

  – Stroke the center of your baby's lower lip with the tip of your nipple. Brush your nipple lightly over the lower lip, as if giving a signal. If you are able, express a few drops of milk to offer a familiar taste and smell. This can also encourage your baby to open his mouth and search for the nipple. When your baby is older and more experienced, this technique of touching your baby's lip with your nipple will be a powerful cue—your baby may open his mouth wide. If he does not open, the lactation specialist or nurse can gently apply slight pressure to his chin to help him open wide or help to shape your nipple and aim it toward the roof of your baby's mouth.

- Then, with a forward movement of the arm encircling your baby, you'll guide him onto your breast. As you do so, aim your nipple up toward the roof of your baby's mouth. This helps ensure you get your nipple above your baby's tongue. Pull him in so close that the tip of his nose touches your breast. Continue to gently compress and support the weight of your breast throughout the *entire* feeding.

Signs That Your Baby Is Properly Latching on to the Breast

- Your baby has a wide-open mouth with lips spread out around your breast.
- Your baby's mouth covers your entire nipple and some of the areola.
- You feel a firm tug on your breast every time your baby sucks.
- Your baby can suckle for more than 3 or 4 sucks in a row.
- Your baby can hang onto your nipple during pauses between bursts of sucks.

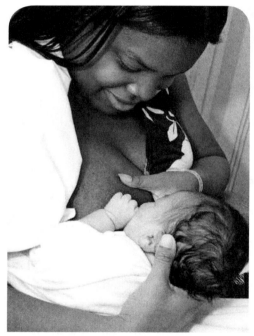

The football or clutch hold works well for many preterm babies. Hold the baby at your side, with his mouth in front of your breast and his feet pointing toward your back. Your opposite hand supports the breast and guides the nipple into the baby's mouth.

Courtesy of Gigi O'Dea.

Is Your Baby Getting Milk?

Once your baby is latched on well, he will suck in small, quick bursts until your milk begins to flow. Then the sucking pattern will change to slower, deeper, more rhythmic sucks. If the NICU is quiet, you may be able to hear your baby swallow. This is a sure sign that he is getting milk. If you cannot hear swallowing, look at his neck for swallowing movement or ask your nurse or lactation specialist to observe you breastfeeding and confirm that your baby is swallowing.

When you first begin to breastfeed, your milk-ejection (letdown) reflex may not occur until after your baby has tired of sucking and fallen asleep. But, just as your body became conditioned to respond to the breast pump, you will learn to respond to your baby's suck.

After a few minutes of sustained, rhythmic sucks, your baby may revert to bursts of little sucks with long pauses in between. The swallowing sounds will be further and further apart. It's time to take your baby off your breast (mothers may need to break the suction with a full-term baby by putting their finger in the baby's mouth to interrupt sucking), burp him, and switch to the other breast. On the second side, watch again for the sucking pattern to slow down and swallowing to become less frequent.

During early feedings, your preterm baby may not be able to tolerate this "burp and switch" technique. Taking your baby off the breast and switching him back and forth may tire him. Ask your lactation specialist for advice about nursing on only one breast at a feeding.

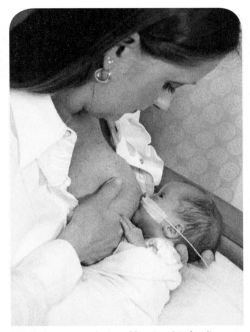

This baby seems alert and begins this feeding at the breast. When he tires, the remainder of the feeding will be given through his gavage tube. *Courtesy of Gigi O'Dea.*

Some NICUs weigh the baby (fully clothed) before and after a feeding to estimate how much milk the baby got during the feeding. Each gram of weight gain is equal to approximately 1 mL of milk. For example, if your baby gained 15 g after a feeding, your baby took about 15 mL (½ oz). If your NICU uses this method to estimate intake, ask your baby's nurse when the process begins.

At first, your baby may be able to breastfeed only once or twice a day. Growing preterm babies become tired and may lose weight if you push them to nurse more than they are able. Continue to pump immediately after each nursing to maintain your milk supply. Although it's tempting to say, "I breastfed the baby, so I don't need to pump," if you don't keep pumping after every breastfeeding, you risk losing your milk supply. As your baby grows, he will start to wake up and show signs that it's time for a feeding. If breastfeeding has been going well for a few days, supplementing breastfeeding with bottle-feeding does not usually interfere with breastfeeding success.

Ensuring Adequate Nutrition

Whether breastfeeding or formula-feeding, most growing preterm babies need additional calories during their hospitalization. When extra protein, vitamins, and minerals are added to your milk, it is called *fortified breast milk*. Special preterm formula can be offered if there is not maternal or donor breast milk available.

Gaining and Growing

After birth, weight gain and growth are closely watched to ensure good nutrition, which affects brain growth and the ability to learn physical, social, and emotional skills (*developmental outcome*). Your NICU team will plot your baby's growth—weight, length, and head circumference changes— on growth charts.

Weight Gain, Length, and Head Circumference

In the nursery, your baby's weight is usually measured in grams. One ounce equals 28 g, although many NICUs count 1 ounce as 30 g for easier calculations. The Appendix contains a chart to help you convert grams to pounds and ounces.

Babies in the NICU are weighed daily or every few days, depending on their health status. After birth, all babies lose some weight. Term babies may lose up to 7% to 10% of their birth weight; preterm babies may lose up to 12% to 15%. For example, if your son is preterm, weighs 1,200 g at birth, and loses 15% of his birth weight, his weight would fall to 1,020 g (15% of 1,200 is 180 g).

Term babies usually lose weight only for the first few days of life. Preterm newborns may lose weight for longer than a few days before starting to gain it back. At first, your baby may not gain weight regularly. His weight may increase on some days, stay the same on others, and occasionally go down. Even when your baby does begin to gain weight regularly, there will be occasional days of no gain or even a slight loss. Because this can be frustrating, most NICU teams assess a baby's average growth by measuring the baby's weight once a week to see the trend in the weight pattern.

Growth Goals

When your baby is stable and can use energy for growth, the average daily expected weight gain is about 15 g for each kilogram of body weight. When your baby is on full feeds, the goal for weight gain is about 15 to 30 g per day or about ½ to 1 ounce per day.

Your baby's body length and head size (*circumference*) are also important and will be measured periodically. Increase in a healthy baby's head circumference usually means brain growth. Overall, the goal is to increase length and head circumference by about 1 cm (a little less than ½ inch) per week.

> After 53 days in the NICU, progress continues slowly but surely, but, unfortunately, with no end in sight. I can't complain much because both girls are doing so well, but I must admit that the long haul is starting to take its toll emotionally. I've always liked the quote: 'If it doesn't kill you, it makes you stronger.' Well, if that's true, I should be one tough cookie by the end of this!
>
> Billie, mother of **Holland** and **Eden**

Taking Care of Yourself

Breastfeeding is a big commitment while your baby is in the NICU and requires a considerable amount of self-care. Your NICU team, including the lactation specialist, may offer more information about ways to make sure you stay healthy during this time in your life. The following information will get you started and may prompt you to think of additional questions for your NICU team.

Diet

Your healthy pregnancy diet should continue after your baby is born. Make good choices, listen to your body, and eat when you're hungry. Include a variety of protein, fat, and carbohydrates. Ask your health care professional if you should continue to take prenatal vitamins or any nutritional supplement. If you have questions about what to eat, ask your health care professional or your baby's nutritionist for suggestions.

Fluids

Drink about 8 glasses of fluid—which should be mostly water—every 24 hours. This is not difficult for most breastfeeding mothers because each time you pump or nurse you will feel thirsty. Drink each time you are thirsty and keep the color of your urine a clear yellow, not cloudy or a dark yellow.

Caffeine

Caffeine, in the form of coffee, tea, and soda, does not usually cause a problem for breastfeeding babies. Some experts recommend limiting daily coffee intake to less than 25 ounces (about 750 mL)—a little more than two 10-ounce cups of coffee per day.

Rest

You need your rest to recover after childbirth, cope with stress, and make milk. Try to nap at least once during the day. You may need to put a special message on your phone and purpose-fully not answer the phone during nap time.

Talk to your lactation specialist about the need to wake up once or twice during the night to pump your breasts. If you let your breasts get full, milk production slows. Failing to pump at night is one of the most common reasons for low milk supply.

Prescription Medications, Over-the-counter Medications, and Herbs

Tell your lactation specialist, your health care professional, and the neonatologist about every prescription medication, every over-the-counter medication (for example, cold remedies, antacids), and any herbs or supplements you take. A few of these, such as medication con-taining codeine, can be unsafe during breastfeeding. As a rule, ask your baby's care provider before you take any medication, herb, or nutritional supplement while providing breast milk for your baby.

Alcohol

Many mothers have questions about drinking alcohol now that pregnancy is over. Possible long-term effects of alcohol in maternal milk remain unknown, especially in preterm babies whose brains are still developing. Because alcohol passes into your milk, consider avoiding alcohol use while your baby is preterm. If you have an occasional alcoholic beverage, limit it to a single drink right after nursing or pumping or expressing milk, and avoid breastfeeding or pumping for 2 hours after the drink.

Drug Use and Cigarettes

Don't be afraid to tell your NICU team if you have issues with street drugs or prescription drug dependence. These all pass through your breast milk to your baby and sometimes pro-duce tragic side effects. Your health care professionals should act as your advocate and refer you to the assistance you need. Your well-being and the health of your baby are their top priorities. Let your team help you find assistance so you can be the best parent possible.

Nicotine and other poisons in cigarettes pass into your breast milk and into your baby. You may have been able to stop smoking during pregnancy, but many parents start again during the NICU stay. Cigarettes expose your baby to secondhand and thirdhand smoke and increase your baby's risk of *sudden infant death syndrome* (*SIDS*). Some methods used to stop smoking (patches, gum, and some medications) can be used safely while breastfeeding. Get help and advice to stop smoking while your baby is in the NICU.

About Marijuana

Marijuana is now legal in some states; however, this does not mean it is safe during breastfeeding. Tetrahydrocannabinol (THC) is the main chemical compound in marijuana and has been found in the feces (poop) of babies whose mothers smoke marijuana, which means THC is absorbed and metabolized by the baby. Tetrahydrocannabinol has been found in levels up to 8-times higher in a mother's breast milk than in the mother's bloodstream. Marijuana passes rapidly to the baby's brain and is also stored for weeks in the baby's fatty tissue. At this time, there is no strong research to evaluate the effects of marijuana on baby brain development, but there is some evidence that exposure to marijuana during critical periods of brain development can affect a child's learning abilities and emotional behaviors. In addition, exposure to secondhand marijuana smoke is associated with risk of SIDS, even though breastfeeding reduces the risk of SIDS. Because marijuana passes into your breast milk, consider abstaining from marijuana use, especially while your preterm baby's brain is still developing.

Breastfeeding Challenges

Breastfeeding can be especially challenging for mothers and babies in the NICU. In the beginning, it may seem like you are participating in the feeding process and your baby is not. This is normal. Give yourself and him time to learn, and ask for help when you encounter problems.

Babies Who Cannot Latch On

A few conditions make it difficult or nearly impossible for a baby to latch on. Babies with abnormal openings (*clefts*) in the roof of their mouth (*palate*) or abnormalities of gum or jawbone may have difficulty latching on and creating suction. Some babies with nervous system or heart abnormalities will not have enough strength or coordination to suck effectively. If your baby has one of these problems, talk with your NICU team.

Nipple Preference

Because bottle-feeding is frequently a component of a baby's nutrition plan in the NICU, parents and staff worry about *nipple preference* or *nipple confusion*. This describes a situation in which a baby develops difficulty with breastfeeding after exposure to bottles. To avoid giving bottles to

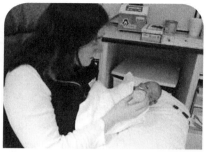

breastfeeding babies, some nurseries use techniques such as finger feeding or cup feeding. With finger feeding, the baby sucks on a gloved finger and a thin feeding tube is slipped into the baby's mouth. With cup feeding, the baby is held upright and small amounts of milk are placed on the baby's tongue with a cup or spoon. These methods have been researched and they do, to some extent, enhance breast-feeding success. If you notice breastfeeding is not going as well after exposure to bottle-feeding, talk about your concern with your NICU team and discuss the various options.

"The feeding and growing stage seemed to go by so slowly."

*Robyn, mother of **Auggie***

Decreasing Milk Supply

You might notice you are producing less milk after the second or third week of pumping. This is less likely to happen if you have a hospital-quality electric pump in good working order, use the double-pumping kit, use breast massage before or during pumping, and are pumping at least 8 times a day. If you skip a pumping session and let your breasts become overly full, your milk

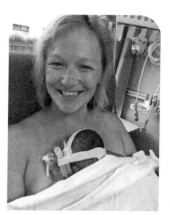

supply will decrease. Pumping frequency is important. Short, frequent pumping (10 minutes, 10 times/day) is better than pumping longer but less often (20 minutes, 5 times/day).

On the other hand, some mothers who pump frequently still have trouble making enough milk and become frustrated when told to pump more often. Feeling anxious or exhausted, not eating or drinking enough, becoming ill, or taking some medications can decrease your milk supply. Ask your NICU team if any drugs you are taking might be affecting your milk supply. Stress reduction and spending more time skin-to-skin with your baby may increase your milk supply. Consider low milk supply a signal to take extra good care of yourself.

Skin-to-skin care is not only good for **Lucy;** it can help increase her mom's milk supply.

Although some recommend various medications or herbal supplements to improve milk supply, there is little scientific evidence on their safety or efficacy. If you are considering trying one of these methods to increase your milk supply, get advice from your lactation specialist and approach this as a team decision.

Sore Nipples

If your nipples become sore from pumping, try turning the pump's suction down, temporarily limiting pumping time to no more than 10 minutes, and applying modified lanolin around the areola before pumping. In addition, you may use a soft, flexible insert made for the electric pump that helps take the pressure off of your sore spot.

Yeast Infection (Thrush)

If your nipples suddenly become sore after being pain-free, or if your nipple pain is not associated with feeding or pumping, you may have a yeast infection. Babies often get an oral yeast infection, called *thrush,* which appears as a milky white coating on the tongue and inner cheeks. Thrush is particularly common in babies who have been on antibiotics. Mothers may develop very sore nipples—which may look perfectly normal or be quite pink—and burning, shooting, or stabbing pains in the breasts. Check your baby's mouth periodically for signs of thrush on the tongue and roof of the mouth.

To treat the yeast infection, you and your baby must be treated together, at the same time. You will need a cream for your nipples, and your baby will receive a liquid medication. During the treatment, you and your baby's caregivers must sterilize pacifiers, breast pump parts, bottle nipples, and anything else that might reinfect your baby's mouth and your breasts. You can continue to breastfeed during treatment. For some mothers, topical treatment alone will not suffice and they will need a 2- to 3-week course of an oral antifungal medication. This medicine is safe to take while breastfeeding or expressing milk for a preterm baby.

Mastitis

If you develop fever and chills, along with a hot, red, tender area on your breast, you probably have a breast infection called *mastitis.* Most cases of mastitis require 2 to 3 weeks of antibiotic treatment. Under ordinary circumstances, women with mastitis and healthy full-term babies should continue to breastfeed or pump; the baby probably has the germ in his mouth already. In the NICU, if your baby has not yet nursed at your breast, your baby's neonatologist may want to discuss the risks and benefits of feeding your breast milk to your baby while you have mastitis.

If you are advised to discard your breast milk while you have mastitis, continue to pump your breasts ("pump and dump") so you can resume breastfeeding as soon as the infection clears up.

Clogged Ducts

A clogged duct produces a red, hot, tender lump on one breast that improves or goes away within about 2 to 3 days. Unlike mastitis, there is no fever. However, if left untreated, it could progress to mastitis.

Treat this problem as if you were coming down with a cold: Take it easy for a couple of days, get enough sleep, and drink extra fluids. In addition, soak your breast several times a day in a tub of warm water, massage it gently (squeezing is painful and not helpful), and pump more frequently. Sometimes, as the clog moves down the duct, a painful white spot develops on the tip of the nipple. This will go away after the clogged duct is clear again.

Clogged ducts are sometimes caused by a mechanical obstruction—for example, an underwire bra that presses in on the breast, a shoulder strap, or your sleep position. Talk to a lactation specialist if you get clogged ducts often.

Too Much Breast Milk

Sometimes, a mother will make so much milk, she is in a position to donate her milk to help other mothers and babies in need. On a much sadder note, a mother who loses her baby may also consider donating her milk. Ask your lactation specialist if there is a milk bank donation center near your home or the hospital. You will need to have your blood tested to make sure you do not have any diseases that could harm another mother's baby. If you meet the donor qualifications, your gift of breast milk can make a big difference in the life of someone else's NICU baby.

If You Need to Stop Breastfeeding

Even under the best of circumstances, not all mothers and babies can breastfeed. It's normal to grieve the loss of something you looked forward to and valued. If you pumped for even a few days, you truly did breastfeed. Your baby will experience some long-lasting health benefits if he received even a little of your milk. If possible, consider donor breast milk for your baby. Your lactation specialist and NICU team can advise you about this.

If you are able to stop breastfeeding over a period of days or a few weeks, your milk supply will gradually diminish and cause little discomfort. But if you have an abundant milk supply and stop breastfeeding suddenly, you may be very uncomfortable. If you experience painfully full breasts when you stop breastfeeding, read ahead to the section titled If You Experience Breast Engorgement.

Bottle-feeding Basics for All NICU Babies

Most preterm babies get breast milk from a bottle while they learn to breastfeed. You may also hear this called "nipple feeding." In any case, parents who are providing breast milk may also need to know the basics of how to feed their baby from a bottle.

Bottles and Nipples

Bottles designed for babies in the NICU usually hold 1½ or 2 ounces, and measurements are marked on the side of the bottle. The NICU staff measure the amount by using the more accurate metric system. One ounce contains about 30 mL. A preterm newborn's first feeding is usually 1 to 2 mL (about ¼ teaspoon).

The nipples for bottles come in a variety of shapes and sizes. Some nipples are smaller and softer, while others are larger and stiffer. The NICU staff will help determine which nipples work best for your baby.

Learning to Bottle-feed

Feeding a baby in the NICU can be challenging. Here are some tips for bottle-feeding your newborn in the NICU. Additional tips for feeding at home are discussed in Chapter 9.

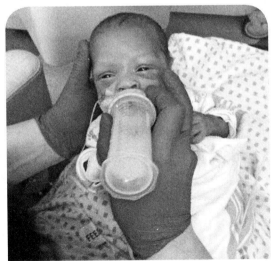

Nathan's first bottle of breast milk.

Watch Your Baby's Feeding Cues

Do what you can to help your baby be alert and ready when you offer the bottle. If you notice preparations for feeding (for example, diapering, dressing) seem to tire your baby, feed him first, straight from the bed. Save the diapering for later. Although some parents prefer to warm formula before feeding, most babies accept room-temperature formula just fine. When feeding breast milk, your nurse or lactation consultant will teach you the correct way to warm breast milk from the refrigerator or freezer.

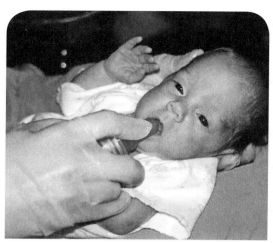

A preterm baby may try to bottle-feed with his tongue on top of the nipple. You can help position the nipple correctly by guiding the nipple, with your finger on top of it, into his mouth.

Position Your Baby Properly

Hold your baby comfortably in your arms and close to your body, with his head slightly raised. If your baby's arms and legs are limp, bend them into a flexed position. Don't sit where bright lights will shine in your baby's face, and take a break if the noise in the NICU becomes too loud. Never prop the bottle. Your baby could choke or could spit up the milk and breathe it back into his lungs (*aspirate*). You may want to alternate the arm that you use to hold your baby during feedings to encourage equal and balanced muscle development in your baby.

Let Your Baby Set the Pace

Relax, and let your baby set the pace during bottle-feeding. Don't try to hurry the process by wiggling and turning and pumping the nipple in your baby's mouth. Forcing milk into a baby's mouth can cause breathing pauses (*apnea*), slow heart rate (*bradycardia*), and *oxygen desaturation*. If the baby can't control the fast flow of milk from the bottle, he may choke or aspirate.

On the other hand, a feeding that lasts longer than 30 minutes may leave your baby exhausted. Often, a baby who successfully finishes part of the feeding will receive the remainder of the feeding through the gavage tube. You will learn to read your baby's cues and follow his pace; he will tell you whether to stop feeding or to continue. This partnership with your baby—this mutual understanding—takes time, but it is basic to successful feeding.

If You Can't Provide Breast Milk

Families feed formula to their babies in the NICU for many different reasons. Sometimes, a mother tries and is unable to produce enough milk, or the baby is not able to breastfeed. Sometimes, medical problems make breastfeeding impossible. Unless there is a medical reason for not breastfeeding, the NICU team will probably encourage you to provide milk or consider using donor breast milk. Consider the pros and cons carefully and make the choice that is right for you and your baby. The NICU staff will support your decision and encourage your active participation in feeding your new baby.

If you feed formula to your baby, ask your baby's nurse about skin-to-skin (kangaroo) care (see Chapter 6). This method of skin-to-skin holding is not just for breastfeeding mothers. Most NICUs encourage both parents to enjoy the skin-to-skin warmth of kangaroo care, and parents appreciate the family closeness it offers. Providing skin-to-skin time with your baby in the NICU is helpful for bonding and establishing caregiving confidence. After you take your baby home, find times to hold him skin-to-skin; for example, after a bath or first thing in the morning. Allow yourself and your baby the pleasure of skin-to-skin contact.

If You Experience Breast Engorgement

After you give birth, your body produces hormones that signal your breasts to make milk. In 2 to 3 days, your breasts swell with milk. If you don't remove the milk by nursing your baby or pumping, your breasts may become rock-hard and painful. The swelling may extend up into your armpits, making even simple movements uncomfortable. You may develop a mild fever. This combination of symptoms is called *engorgement*.

After 2 or 3 days of engorgement, you'll notice your breasts are getting softer and more comfortable. If you are not breastfeeding, they will return to their prepregnancy size in several weeks. Until then, you may notice milk leaking from the nipples. Some women who do not breastfeed (or stop breastfeeding) notice leaking for several months. This is normal, but leaking can be prolonged by anything that causes nipple stimulation—for example, running or other exercise that causes your breasts to bounce and any stimulation that involves your breasts and nipples. If you still have milk 6 to 12 months after giving birth, or if you think the leaking is excessive (and you've tried reducing the amount of nipple stimulation), talk to your health care professional.

Managing Breast Engorgement

While you wait for the engorgement to resolve naturally, try these comfort measures.

- If you do not plan to breastfeed, use a breast pump or hand express just enough milk to relieve the pressure. You can discard the milk or ask the hospital staff for containers so it can be given to your baby for these few days. As the swelling subsides, gradually pump or express less often. In a few days, you'll be able to stop altogether.

- Apply cold compresses, such as gel packs made for this purpose, a bag of frozen peas, wet washcloths chilled in the freezer, or the classic Australian remedy of cold raw cabbage leaves.

- Wear a bra if it fits well and feels good. If you have a sports bra, try that. Wear it to bed if the pain is keeping you awake at night.

- Take a pain reliever recommended by your health care professional.

- Try heat to relieve the pain. Wrap your breasts in warm, wet washcloths (covered with plastic wrap to keep the heat in), or take a warm shower, allowing any milk produced to flow down the drain.

Your Baby Needs You

· · · · · · · · · · · · ·

Feeding is a common area of concern for the families of full-term and preterm babies, for parents of babies who are healthy at birth and for those who need intensive care. Not only is nourishment vital to your baby's well-being, but feeding is closely related to many other areas of your baby's care and healthy future. Whatever your concerns, questions, or struggles, specialists in the NICU will help you find the best answers.

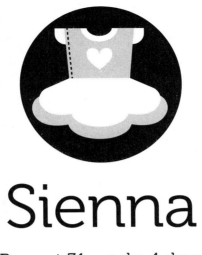

Sienna

Born at 31 weeks 4 days

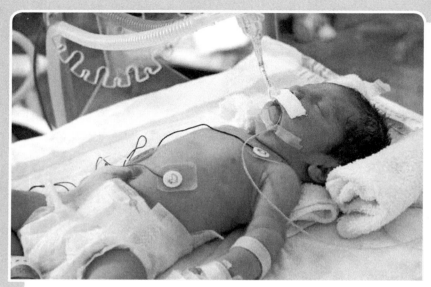

Sienna soon after birth.

Sienna was born at 31 weeks 4 days of gestation, after a placental abruption caused her premature birth. She spent her first 19 days in the NICU, learning to breathe and eat on her own. I lived about 45 minutes away from the hospital, so every day I drove there, spent the day, and tearfully departed for home in the late hours of the evening. In the beginning, I knew it was necessary and Sienna had to be under their care and supervision.

The doctors and nurses provided incredible care for her in those early, fragile days, and for that, I could not possibly be more grateful. Sienna proved, very early on, that she was a fighter and did not plan to stay there for too long. Within a few days, she was breathing on her own and out of the incubator. She spent the majority of her stay learning how to eat on her own, without a feeding tube. Every day, Sienna progressed little by little.

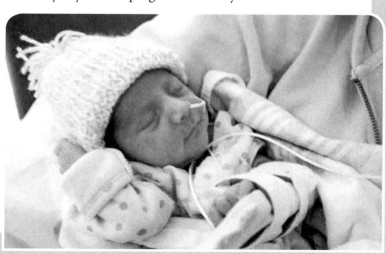

Sienna making progress.

When she was finally able to come home, my heart was full of happiness but also anxiety, as she would no longer be hooked up to sensors that would alarm to tell me something was off. Thankfully, the transition from NICU to home was seamless.

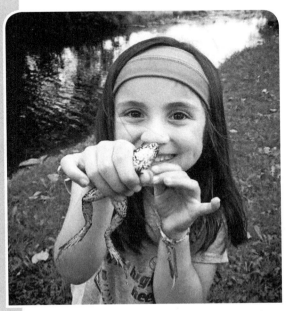

"Sienna at 5 years old in this photo. She loves to be outside! This was her first time catching a frog. She is fearless and brave."

Kaitlynn, mother of Sienna

Today, Sienna is 6 years old. She has no health problems and no development issues. She is incredibly smart and one of the strongest readers in her class. She was blessed with artistic talent, as well as a great left-handed shot with her bow and arrow. She has a beautiful, giving, and compassionate heart to go along with her resilient "tough girl" attitude. I believe that Sienna's entrance into this world was one that was predestined in order to shape her into the sweet, smart, and healthy little girl that she is today. She makes my heart soar and has given me purpose in life.

Kaitlynn, mother of Sienna

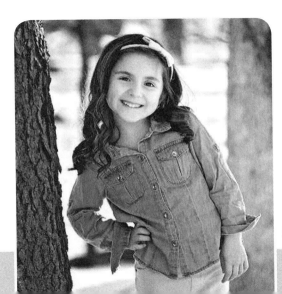

Sienna, at age 6 years.

CHAPTER 8

Homeward Bound

"There was so much anticipation and buildup for our son's discharge from the NICU that by the time the day arrived, I was surprised by my sudden sadness to leave the place I so desperately wanted to flee."

*Robyn, mother of **Auggie***

As your baby grows and the most serious medical problems begin to resolve, you will start thinking about getting ready to bring your baby home. During this phase of your baby's hospital stay, there is generally a greater focus on parent involvement. Learning to care for your baby becomes the focal point of time spent with your baby.

The Intermediate Care Experience

Some babies go home directly from the neonatal intensive care unit (NICU), but some are moved to a less intensive environment, sometimes called a "step-down unit." One day, your NICU team may tell you, "It's graduation day! Your baby is leaving the NICU and moving to the intermediate care nursery. It won't be long now until you can take your baby home."

Graduation sounds like progress (and it is!), but what else changes? Being a NICU parent has meant dealing with daily changes, but by now you have developed a comfort level with the NICU staff, equipment, routines, and procedures. Things may be different in the new unit. This change means another period of adjustment.

The step-down unit may be within the NICU itself or very nearby. Some NICUs transfer babies to a community hospital closer to home and, maybe, where your NICU journey first began. Knowing what to expect in the way of routines, staff members, and your role during this period will help you feel more comfortable and learn what you'll need to know when your baby comes home.

Transferring to a Step-down Unit

If your baby is transferred to a step-down unit, it may be called *intermediate care, NICU step-down, special care nursery, growing preemie unit, Level II unit,* or something else. Whatever the unit is called, your baby's transfer means he has passed the need for intensive medical care. With a few exceptions, your baby is past the major medical problems and is on the road home.

As your NICU team prepares you for this new phase of care, they may describe the intermediate care setting as a quieter place, more able to work with your baby's sleep/wake cycles and abilities to interact with his less hectic surroundings. Because growing babies need a lot of undisturbed

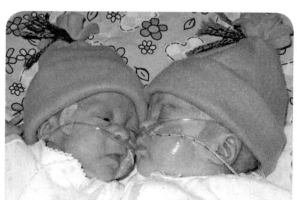

"The good news is that on Sunday, we moved to a different room in the NICU for kids who need less critical care. I guess you could say we 'graduated'! **Eden** weighs 4 pounds 6 ounces, and **Holland** weighs 3 pounds 11.5 ounces. It's looking hopeful that we will be home by Thanksgiving."

*Billie, mother of **Holland** and **Eden***

rest, feeding time is often the best time for interaction; therefore, your team may suggest you spend this time with your baby, learning about his emerging personality, cues, and behaviors.

Your baby no longer requires frequent intensive nursing care, so expect his nurse to be caring for 2 to 3 other babies. Depending on the hospital, the nursing staff in the intermediate care setting may be the same as the NICU, and you may even have the same primary nurse. In many hospitals, your baby's doctors and consulting specialists will remain the same in the new setting. Occupational or physical therapists may work with you and your baby more frequently now on feeding skills, positioning, comforting, and other behavioral and physical tasks.

Transferring to a Community Hospital

If your baby was transferred to the NICU from another hospital, your NICU team may discuss transporting him back to your community hospital for continued convalescence and preparation for discharge. *Back transport*—also called *return transport*—is common in hospitals where NICU beds are used for the sickest babies and less intensive care is done in community hospital special care nurseries. The community hospital is often closer to your home and may allow you to spend more time with your baby.

Community hospitals with special care nurseries are pleased and excited to care for your baby. You may discover that you can learn to care for your baby in a more relaxed setting and also receive more individual attention. People who can help you and your baby make the transition to home are available at the community hospital and are very familiar with local support sources, such as medical equipment supply companies and community home health services. If your baby requires complex care, you can ask what access the community nursery has to specialty staff— such as neurologists, ophthalmologists, and pulmonologists—for consultations.

Becoming Comfortable in New Surroundings

If your baby moves to an intermediate care nursery or community hospital that has a different staff, you may miss the comfortable working relationships you shared with the NICU staff. You and your baby may need some time to get acquainted with a new team and learn how to communicate well with that team. Eventually, you will develop good communication and trusting relationships with staff members in the intermediate care nursery, just as you did with those in the NICU.

You may need to adjust to new routines and procedures. One of the biggest challenges of becoming comfortable in a new setting is understanding that *different* is not necessarily *wrong*. In addition to learning about the new unit routines, communicate your baby's likes and dislikes, including his typical behavior patterns, with the staff. They will be most appreciative of the information during this period when everyone is getting acquainted.

Emotional Changes

As things slow down, you may find that emotions from the past weeks are catching up with you. You may have been too frightened or overwhelmed to express some of those feelings, but now they seem to come tumbling out at your partner, the nursery staff, and anyone else who is willing to listen. This is common and will slow down eventually.

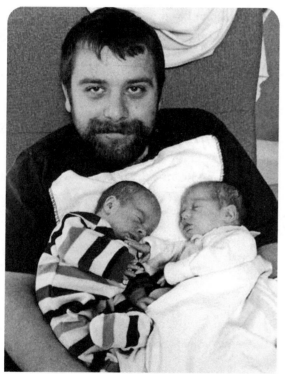

If your anxiety does not decrease, or if you are having trouble sleeping or eating or taking care of your daily needs, tell your doctor or your baby's social worker or nurse. They can help you find resources before your baby is ready to come home.

Adjusting to the Change

The transfer process is a lot of activity for a preterm baby. He may be sleepier than usual or may not tolerate feedings well for the first 24 hours in the new environment. Some babies require a slight increase in supplemental oxygen following a transport, or they might lose a bit of weight for the first few days. Given an opportunity for quiet rest, your baby will quickly recover and adapt to this new setting.

Preparing for discharge can be almost as stressful as your first days in the NICU. Matthew spends some relaxing quiet time with twins **Bailey Jo** and **Abraham** as discharge day approaches.

*Matthew, father of **Bailey Jo** and **Abraham***

Your Expanding Role in Care

During this phase of the hospital stay, you and your baby will master the skills necessary for discharge. This is the time to take a more active role in your baby's care.

As discharge nears, you'll need the nurse's help less often. Your baby's nurse may still talk you through more complex tasks, but by now you should be fairly comfortable taking a temperature or changing a diaper. Use your nurse as a resource whenever you have questions or need assistance during this learning period.

What Do You Need to Know?

You'll need to know your baby's schedule to participate in care. Ask about the feeding schedule, bath time, and special treatments, such as respiratory or physical therapy. Let the nurses know what you feel comfortable doing (for example, changing a diaper) and what skills you're ready to learn (such as giving vitamins). Nurses will gladly save a feeding or bath for parents or rearrange your baby's schedule to fit your schedule if this is discussed ahead of time. The intermediate care nursery also provides an excellent opportunity to begin or continue skin-to-skin (kangaroo) care.

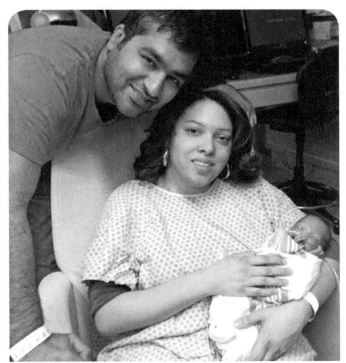

With many of his medical issues behind him, **Nathan** gains weight and improves his feeding skills in this phase of his NICU journey.

Hands-on Skills You Will Need Before Discharge

- Feeding
- Diapering
- Dressing
- Taking a temperature
- Bathing
- Giving medication
- How to use any medical devices your baby will need after discharge
- Infant cardiopulmonary resuscitation (CPR)

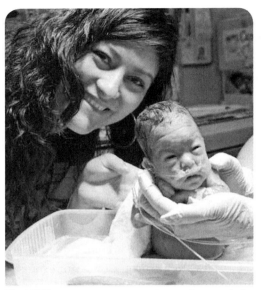

The NICU team encourages you to care for your baby as soon as you and the baby are ready. This mother is learning to bathe her baby.

Courtesy of University of Washington Medical Center, Seattle, WA.

Jack has graduated to an open crib. Maintaining a normal body temperature in a crib while still gaining weight is a big step toward going home.

Milestones a Preterm Baby Will Meet Before Discharge

- He needs to have "outgrown" his apnea, bradycardia, and desaturation episodes.
- He needs to show a regular trend of weight gain on the feeding plan that is in place.
- He needs to maintain a normal temperature in an open crib.

> "Holland taught Mommy a good lesson today on diaper changing. Lesson: One must wait to change the diaper until the baby is finished going...3 diapers later and all-new bedding and we were back on track!"
>
> Billie, mother of **Holland** and **Eden**

Common Health Issues During This Phase

Now that your baby is in the "feeding and growing" phase of NICU care, he is past many of the dangers that may have been present while he was critically ill. As your baby approaches hospital discharge, here are some common health issues that may still require attention.

Bronchopulmonary Dysplasia

If your preterm baby has bronchopulmonary dysplasia (also called *chronic lung disease*), he may still require breathing support, additional oxygen, and medications. As oral feeding progresses, your baby may have some days that he needs more oxygen and does not breathe as comfortably. These ups and downs are normal but can be very frustrating. During this phase of care, your NICU team will determine if support can be weaned before hospital discharge or if your baby will still need some type of breathing support at home.

Apnea and Bradycardia

Apnea, bradycardia, and desaturations are a common problem for preterm babies, and these events may continue during this phase. Unless they are a side effect of another illness, these events go away as your baby's brain matures and almost always vanish before your baby's original due date. The staff will monitor the frequency, intensity, and duration of the episodes. If medication is used to control apnea, it may be stopped before hospital discharge and your baby will continue to use a cardiac monitor for a period of time to ensure that the medication is no longer needed. Sometimes, waiting for apnea and bradycardia to resolve is the final step before a baby is ready for discharge.

Gastroesophageal Reflux

A condition known as *gastroesophageal reflux* (*GER*) occurs when swallowed milk moves back up the food pipe (*esophagus*). A baby with GER might spit up frequently and lose a lot of what he eats. He may have signs of discomfort during feeding and poor weight gain. Gastroesophageal reflux can be frustrating for parents and caregivers. Some babies will improve with frequent burping, adjusting the head of the bed, changing the baby's position during or after feeding, changing the feeding, or changing the baby's formula if the baby is not receiving breast milk. There is no scientific evidence showing that any treatment significantly improves GER. Many preterm babies show symptoms of GER, and most babies outgrow it as they reach their original due date. In some cases, consultation with a gastrointestinal specialist may be needed to help resolve this problem.

Anemia

Growing preterm babies frequently have anemia of prematurity (low red blood cell [RBC] count). Recall that anemia of prematurity occurs because RBC production temporarily stops after birth (see Chapter 5). The amount of RBCs, measured by the hemoglobin level, reaches its lowest value between 4 and 10 weeks after birth.

If your baby still requires additional oxygen, he may need occasional blood transfusions. If your baby is stable and growing well, the nursery team may allow the hemoglobin level to drop to stimulate his own RBC production system. In addition, growing preterm babies may receive extra iron to support blood cell production. In some hospitals, a medication will be given to stimulate RBC production. If your baby still has anemia at the time of discharge, your pediatrician may continue to check his blood cell count until it starts to increase.

Hernias

Preterm babies are at risk for hernias—when a loop of intestine moves through a muscle weakness or other opening inside the body.

Inguinal Hernia

The most common hernia is called an *inguinal hernia*. This condition occurs most often in boys and usually presents as a bulge in the groin, especially after crying or straining during a bowel movement. Sometimes girls get inguinal hernias, which cause a bulge, or swelling, above or along the labia (near the vaginal opening).

A boy's testicles are inside the abdomen during development and stay high in the groin (*inguinal canal*) until about 32 weeks' gestation. At that time, the testicles descend through the canal into the scrotum. In preterm babies, part of the intestine may also push through the canal into the scrotum. This may affect one or both sides and appears as a swelling above or in the scrotum.

As long as the intestine can be easily and gently pushed back through the opening (the hernia is *reducible*), immediate surgical correction is not necessary. Surgery to repair the hernia may occur before discharge, or it may be delayed until your baby is older. If the intestine becomes trapped in the groin or scrotum (*incarcerated hernia*), the skin overlying the hernia or the scrotum will become swollen, blue, and painful, and immediate surgery is necessary.

Umbilical Hernia

Another area where a hernia can occur is around the umbilical area or belly button. In this case, the ring of muscle and supporting tissue at the base of the belly button is loose and allows a loop of intestine to push outward when the baby cries. As long as there is no redness or discoloration, there is no cause for concern. A small *umbilical hernia* often corrects itself as your baby grows and the abdominal muscles strengthen and thicken. In general, surgical correction is not recommended before the age of 3 to 5 years.

Predischarge Testing

While you're learning all you can about your baby's care, the health care team is planning your baby's final tests and making preparations for discharge. Common discharge tests are explained here, but not all babies require all of the tests discussed, and some may have even more. Ask your baby's team what to expect as discharge draws near.

Eye Examination

If your baby was 30 weeks' gestation or less or weighed less than 1,500 g (3 lb 5 oz) at birth, he will have an eye examination between 4 and 7 weeks of age. Babies born after 30 weeks' gestation and weighing between 1,500 and 2,000 g may also have this type of eye examination if they were particularly sick in the newborn period. Follow-up examinations will be scheduled if necessary. The examination is to identify any changes in the eye tissue caused by retinopathy of prematurity (see Chapter 5).

Hearing Test

Using electronic sound and response monitoring, automated hearing tests—also called *audiology screenings*—are used to help determine if your baby hears normally. Environmental conditions, such as surrounding noise or a crying baby, can cause inconclusive results. If this happens, a repeat test will be planned when your baby is sleeping and the room is quieter. After discharge, your child's hearing should be monitored by your pediatrician at periodic health examinations. If you are concerned about your baby's hearing, alert your pediatrician so additional testing can be scheduled if necessary.

> ❝ Pascal weaned off his high-flow nasal cannula, finished his antibiotics, and then failed his car seat test, then again, then again. You know those 5 stages of grief? I was stuck oscillating between acceptance and bargaining: 'If he's not safe to go home, then we'll stay, of course we'll stay. But we don't live very far! I can get a different stroller that doesn't take the car seat! The kind with the bassinet! I won't leave him in bouncy seats!' Each time, the nurse or the fellow would talk me through it: 'He's not safe to go home. He just needs more time.' ❞
>
> Alex, father of **Pascal**

Car Safety Seat Trial

Ask your health care team if your baby will have a *car safety seat trial* (sometimes called an *angle tolerance test*) before discharge. The American Academy of Pediatrics (AAP) recommends this

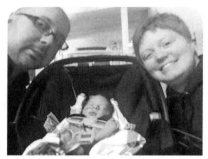

Maxwell is positioned correctly in his car seat for his car safety seat trial. Note the pulse oximeter on Maxwell's foot, which helps determine if Maxwell can tolerate this position without bradycardia or desaturation.

evaluation if your baby is born preterm or has certain other medical problems. During a car safety seat trial, your baby is positioned in the car seat you bought and his heart rate, breathing, and oxygen saturation are monitored for a period of time. For tips about purchasing a car safety seat, see the Car Safety Seat section later in this chapter. The car safety seat trial helps to determine if your baby can tolerate the upright position of the car safety seat without having breathing problems. If he has apnea, bradycardia, or desaturations in the car seat, the team may suggest a different type of car safety seat that allows the baby to lie flat while traveling (*car bed*), investigate other problems, or delay your discharge to allow your baby to grow. They may also advise you to avoid the use of an infant carrier, baby seat, or swing until he is older and stronger.

Pulse Oximetry Screen for Critical Congenital Heart Defects

Most healthy newborns are screened for *critical congenital heart defects* (CCHDs) before they are discharged from the hospital. Critical congenital heart defects are life-threatening and not always diagnosed before birth or in the first few days of life. The screening does not detect all forms of

CCHD, but it is considered a valuable detection tool because an apparently healthy newborn who goes home with an undetected CCHD may be critically ill by the time parents notice signs of trouble and get the baby to an emergency department.

To conduct the screening examination, a pulse oximeter is placed on the right hand and on either foot. If oxygen saturation is at least 95% in both the hand and foot, the baby has "passed" the screening and no further action is necessary. If oxygen saturation is less than 90% in either extremity, the reading is 90% to 94%, or there is a notable difference between the 2 readings despite several attempts, the baby has "failed" the screening. This does not mean the newborn has a heart defect, but the baby should be evaluated further, which includes having an echocardiogram before discharge.

This screening is targeted toward healthy newborns and is not always performed on babies who have been in the NICU. This is because many babies who have been in the NICU have already had an echocardiogram, and others have had their oxygen saturation levels monitored for extended periods, which would reveal a congenital heart defect. The AAP recommends pulse oximetry screening for CCHDs prior to discharge (and after weaning from supplemental oxygen) for any baby who has not had an echocardiogram performed as part of his care.

Immunizations

If your infant is in the hospital for 60 days or more, your baby's doctor will talk to you about the immunizations routinely given at that time. These are the same vaccines your infant would receive in the doctor's office at a 2-month checkup and are important for your baby's health.

Immunizations for Your Baby

With few exceptions, the immunization schedule for preterm infants is the same as that for term infants. You don't have to correct for how early your baby was born. The first dose of hepatitis vaccine that is usually given right after birth may have been delayed, and your baby may need to "catch up." In addition, the rotavirus vaccine is a live virus vaccine; it may not be given until your baby is ready to leave the hospital, or it may be given in your pediatrician's office.

If your infant was very preterm or has significant heart disease, he may be at increased risk of rehospitalization due to *respiratory syncytial virus* (*RSV*) infection. Your doctor will determine if your baby should receive a medication that can decrease this risk. This medication, called palivizumab (brand name Synagis), is given as an injection once a month for 1 to 5 months during the winter.

> At a certain point, after another car seat test failure, his nurse decided we would do something fun, and she set up everything we needed for a bath and instructed me in how to wash him. I did not actually know how to bathe a baby, and to this day, I remain grateful for her teaching and for the photo she took of me bathing him. As a solo parent, it's remarkably hard to get photos of you and the baby together that's not a selfie, and as great as selfies are, there's something sweet about having both my hands in the photo, cradling him in the sink.
>
> Alex, father of **Pascal**

Immunizations for Parents and Family

Immunizing your baby is an important investment in his health and protects him from rehospitalization, but your new baby is not the only one who needs immunizations. Be sure your other children and the adults in your home are up-to-date on all of their immunizations. Ask whether you or other family members need a whooping cough (*pertussis*) booster immunization. Everyone older than 6 months in your family and everyone who will take care of your baby should also receive the influenza vaccine before flu season starts each year. By immunizing yourself, your children, and your baby's caregivers, you are protecting your baby until he is old enough to receive all of his own immunizations.

> John and I are so excited about getting our babies home...but also very nervous. They are going to be very susceptible to colds and other sickness, so we need to be diligent about keeping them as protected as possible. As much as we love company (and all our family and friends), we probably won't be able to see much of anybody. We will be pretty much homebound for much of the winter. We look forward to more visitors this spring!
>
> Billie, mother of **Holland** and **Eden**

Getting What Your Baby Will Need

While your baby is growing stronger and getting ready to go home, it's time to pull out all of the baby care books that you hid away because they seemed so irrelevant to your NICU experience. Look over the baby supply and home preparation lists and start getting what you'll need. Now may also be the time to cue eager friends or family members who have been waiting for the right moment to give you a baby shower.

Shop Wisely

Some baby care items that sound like a good idea are totally unnecessary. For example, do not buy baby sleep positioners that are supposed to keep your baby correctly positioned for safe sleep. If your baby needs a positioner, it will be recommended by your baby's physical therapist. You do not need to buy extra pads or positioners to place in your baby's car safety seat. If it did not come with the seat, and if you did not use it during your baby's safety seat trial in the hospital, do not use it. Remember to ask your NICU team about any questions you may have about baby care items.

Clothing and Diapers

By the time they are ready for discharge, many preterm babies fit into newborn-sized clothes. You may decide to purchase a few "going out" items in preemie size for special occasions, but keep in mind that your baby will quickly outgrow them and seldom use them.

Newborn diapers generally work fine for most preterm babies at discharge. Some hospitals send a small supply of preemie diapers home with you. If necessary, you can buy extra-small diapers online or in many grocery stores and drugstores.

You may begin with a preference for cloth or disposable diapers. But as your baby grows, you may change your mind and decide to use a combination of cloth and disposable supplies.

Breastfeeding Aids

If you have been breastfeeding your baby, you will have the basic supplies already. Most breastfeeding mothers of NICU graduates also need to continue to use a hospital-grade electric breast pump at home for a while after their baby's hospital discharge.

What Does a Baby Need at Home?

Clothing

4–6 T-shirts

8 sleep gowns

6 one-piece T-shirts with snaps at waist or crotch

2–4 sweatshirts or sweaters

1 or 2 outfits for special occasions

6 pairs of booties or socks

12 fabric diaper covers if using cloth diapers

5-dozen cloth diapers (may also be used as burp
    cloths) or disposable diapers

Seasonal

Coat, knit hat

Cotton hat or bonnet

Bedtime

2–3 sleep sacks (no blankets in the crib)

4–6 receiving blankets

6–12 lap pads

2–4 crib sheets

2 waterproof pads (goes under the crib sheet)

Nursery monitor (if you want to use one)

Nightlight

Bath Time

1–2 large hooded towels

2–4 washcloths

Plastic bathtub

Foam bathtub liner (foam bath pillow)

Brush and comb set

Baby shampoo

Baby scissors

Health Care Supplies

Digital thermometer and lubricant

Infant acetaminophen as recommended by your
    baby's health care professional

Medicine dropper

Baby journal and calendar

Furniture

Bassinet or cradle (if baby's sleep location varies)

Crib and mattress or portable crib

Chest of drawers

Laundry hamper

Diaper pail for cloth diapers

Outings

Diaper bag or backpack

Car safety seat

Stroller appropriate to your baby's needs

Breastfeeding

2 or 3 nursing bras

Nursing pads

Hospital-grade electric breast pump

Containers and labels for breast milk storage

Bottle-feeding

8 four-ounce or 8-ounce bottles and nipples

Bottle brush or dishwasher cage

Formula Feeding

Baby formula recommended by your baby's health
    care professional

Miscellaneous

2 or 3 pacifiers (if your baby uses one)

Baby toys and books

Baby memory book

Baby care books

Baby laundry soap

Later

Front carrier or backpack

Baby swing

High chair

Bibs

Feeding spoons and cups

Childproofing supplies

Breast Milk Supplements and Formula

Find out if your baby will be discharged with a breast milk supplement or preterm discharge formula. Talk to your care team and discuss if there is a particular brand you need to purchase or if different brands are interchangeable. Find which store in your area sells the supplement or formula you need. Large retail stores may stock preterm discharge formulas, but smaller stores may need to order them. If your baby requires a special formula, your local pharmacy may need to order it for you. Talk to your discharge planner, dietitian, or social worker to see if the supplement or formula you need is covered by insurance or the government-funded Women, Infants, and Children (WIC) program.

If you used a formula in the hospital, it was most likely provided in a ready-to-feed, premixed bottle. Ready-to-feed formula is convenient, but it is the most expensive. You may want to keep a couple of bottles of ready-to-feed formula in your diaper bag for emergencies during travel. After discharge, you may choose to buy formula as a liquid concentrate or powder that you will mix with water. Talk to your NICU team about which type they recommend. Powder is the least expensive but has a greater risk of becoming contaminated with bacteria. In any case, make sure you carefully follow the instructions for mixing formula provided by your doctor and dietitian.

Water from most public water systems is acceptable for infant use. To be sure, however, ask your baby's NICU team about the necessity of boiling supplies when preparing formula, including the water used to dilute concentrate or powder formula. Most physicians are comfortable with a thorough washing of all supplies with hot soapy water and a bottle brush. Most dishwashers are also efficient for bottle washing. If you have an alternate water source, such as a well, or if lead or naturally high fluoride levels in the water are a concern, check with your baby's NICU team or the public health department for its recommendations.

Car Safety Seat

A car safety seat is also called a child safety seat or child restraint. It doesn't matter what term you use—the fact remains that using a car safety seat every time your baby is in the car is one of the most important things you can do to protect him. Many parents convince their children when they are very young that the car engine will not start until every person is buckled up. This routine may also offer an opportunity to convince other family members of the importance of using seat belts.

It's very important to place your baby in an approved car safety seat when you take him anywhere in a vehicle. In all 50 states, car safety seat use is mandated by law. Each year, thousands of infants and young children are killed or injured in car crashes. Proper use of car safety seats helps keep children safe. Your lap is never a safe place for your baby in a moving vehicle. If your baby needs your attention and can't wait until you reach your destination, pull over and stop the car in a safe place to help him. Car safety seats should be used only for travel and never for sleeping or feeding.

All babies need to use a car safety seat that fits their weight, height, and any special needs. If your baby weighs less than 5 pounds, check that the seat's manufacturer allows it to be used for babies at your child's weight. Some seats come with an additional insert that helps very small babies fit better, but parents should only use inserts that came in the box with the seat and never use any other product inside the car safety seat. Babies with certain medical conditions may need to use a different kind of restraint known as a *car bed*. Before the anticipated discharge date, you will bring your baby's car safety seat to the hospital and a member of the care team will monitor your baby's heart rate, breathing, and oxygen saturation to see if the baby's semi-upright position in the car safety seat causes any problems.

Most car safety seats are not installed correctly in the car; if your hospital does not have a certified car safety seat technician on staff who can help you, you can find a certified technician at **http://cert.safekids.org** or by calling the National Highway Traffic Safety Administration Vehicle Safety Hotline at 888/327-4236. This should be done before your baby is discharged from the NICU so you can insure the car safety seat is correctly installed into your car. Readers may want to visit the official AAP Web site for parents at **www.HealthyChildren.org/carseatguide** to keep current on this topic.

Stroller

A stroller is valuable for carrying not only your baby, but all of your baby supplies. If your baby requires special medical equipment, purchase the best-manufactured stroller you can afford. Compare brands, and talk to other parents of babies with special needs before deciding. Look for safety features, sturdiness, storage space, and ease in collapsing and setting up. Umbrella strollers and most baby backpacks and carriers do not give adequate support for young babies.

Nursery Monitor

Different from a cardiac monitor, a nursery monitor is an intercom and, sometimes, a video camera that helps you hear or see your baby in his crib from wherever you are in the house. If you choose to purchase a monitor, look closely at the listening range, power requirements, and ease of use. Remember that your baby monitor may pick up signals from other baby monitors in your neighborhood, and your neighbors' baby monitors may be able to pick up everything happening in your baby's room. Purchase one with more than one channel to decrease the risk of interference with your other electronic devices.

To keep your baby safe from accidental injury—for example, strangulation by the nursery monitor cord or electrical shock from putting parts in his mouth—be sure to place the base of the monitor and other accessories out of your baby's reach, and never take this equipment near water, such as in the bathroom.

Bulletin Board, Calendar, and Journal

A bulletin board, calendar, or journal is not on most baby supply lists, but some parents of NICU graduates must keep track of a multitude of appointments and information. Consider posting important information, such as names and contact information for your health care team, appointments, developmental milestones, medication schedules, and instructions from your physical therapist, on a bulletin board or in a journal. Figure out what will work best for you and your partner. This will become your "communication station"—especially if your baby's care needs are complex. Some parents use a smartphone, notebook, or tablet, which can be taken to medical appointments, to keep track of this information as well. Having one place for all of this important information will be extremely helpful when getting organized.

> Regardless of how much time you're able to spend in the NICU, make it count. Put your phone away, hold your baby skin to skin, and get to know your baby. This helps you build a strong bond, it helps you learn about your baby's personality and moods and patterns, and it prepares you for life outside the NICU.
>
> Kate and Matthew, parents of **Lucy**

Arranging for Medical and Other Care After Discharge

Your baby is making good progress toward a homecoming date. You've purchased supplies and equipment, and you're comfortable with most of your baby's care tasks. Before your baby is discharged from the hospital, you need to arrange for his continuing medical care.

Choosing Your Baby's Health Care Professional

Parents are sometimes caught the week before their baby's discharge without a clue as to who will provide their baby's care. If you have not yet chosen a pediatrician, begin the interviewing process well before discharge. Finding a new doctor can be an unsettling experience, especially after you've come to know and trust the hospital staff. As with any new relationship, expect a time of adjustment, uncertainty, and nervousness until trust is established. You need time to get acquainted.

Most neonatologists do not see infants outside the NICU or intermediate care unit, but, depending on where you live, they may be able to recommend a pediatric practice in your area. It would be a good idea to get recommendations for a new pediatrician weeks before discharge. Your insurance program may have a list of pediatricians; bring the list to the NICU for help developing a list of potential candidates. Nurses, close friends, or parents of NICU graduates are other possible sources of recommendations. If you do not have access to a pediatrician where you live, a healthy NICU graduate may be cared for by a family physician or qualified pediatric nurse practitioner. After you have a few names in hand, call and schedule a "meet the doctor" visit. Ask if this visit is free of charge or covered by your insurance because some offices will charge for this time. As you interview potential candidates, keep in mind that personality type and coping styles—yours and the doctor's—play a large part in the decision. Questions to ask are included in the "'Meet the Doctor' Interview Questions" box.

Babies with special needs should have one doctor who is able to follow their progress. Choosing a pediatrician before your baby is discharged allows the neonatologist or primary physician caring for your baby to speak directly with the pediatrician or to send the doctor a written discharge summary of your baby's hospital course. If at all possible, your baby should be seen by a consistent physician rather than at a general health unit or clinic, where medical personnel change often. Many pediatricians accept patients on public assistance if you are without private insurance. In some states, Medicaid will also provide transportation for you to take your baby to the doctor.

Your pediatrician will become an important resource person as your NICU graduate continues to grow and develop. The pediatrician you choose should be trained in the care of infants and children with special conditions, such as preterm birth, or special needs, such as technology dependence.

"Meet the Doctor" Interview Questions

- Where do you have hospital privileges? If our baby requires readmission to the hospital, will you be the primary doctor or will you refer to a hospitalist or a specialist?
- Is this your primary office location? Do you have other "satellite" offices near my home?
- What are your office hours?
- Do you do laboratory testing in your office, or do we need to drive to another location?
- How would I schedule an appointment?
- Who is available to answer baby care questions during the day? After hours?
- How far in advance do I need to call for an appointment?
- How is billing handled?
- Do you care for other babies with histories similar to my baby? What is your training and experience with a baby like mine?
- Will other clinicians in your practice see my baby? May I meet them today?
- What procedure do we follow if we need you on a weekend or at night?
- How do we handle emergencies—should we call you first or go directly to the emergency department?
- Do you offer parent education classes?

Establishing a Medical Home

A *medical home* is a concept of care that means families and health care professionals work together to coordinate all of a child's care. It means having a home base for health care focused on the whole child, not just one part. In a medical home, you are valued as the expert in your child's care and treated as an important member of your child's health care team.

Your baby may go home with ongoing special health care needs. You may need help locating resources, getting referrals, making appointments, and coordinating your baby's care with several health care professionals. The doctor in your baby's medical home will be your guide during this process, helping to identify, access, and coordinate all of the medical and nonmedical services your baby needs.

Understanding Referrals

Certain specialists may continue to follow your baby after discharge. The neonatologist may call the specialist to discuss your baby's hospital course and arrange for a copy of the discharge summary to be sent to the specialist's office. Some specialists may prefer to see your baby in the hospital before discharge. The consulting physician will usually meet with you or talk with you on the phone. He or she will indicate when and where follow-up examinations should occur. It is very important to attend these follow-up appointments as scheduled.

You should ask for a copy of your baby's discharge summary. Keeping a copy of this summary is helpful in case you change doctors or have to see other specialists. If your baby has complex medical problems, keep one in your diaper bag so you have the information handy in case of emergency. If you have questions about anything you read in the summary, ask your baby's doctor or nurse practitioner.

> **Both girls are becoming much more social lately and are waking up more to look around, especially when I'm there. Got to hold both of them tonight for a good cuddle!**
>
> Billie, mother of **Holland** and **Eden**

Decisions to Make as Discharge Nears

If many miles have separated you from your baby, now is the time to use any available resources to spend as much time as possible with him before discharge. Ask your discharge planner for help with this very important aspect of parent education. But whether you're close to your baby's hospital or far away, you still need to make more decisions and preparations before your baby comes home. Ask your NICU social worker about facilities such as the Ronald McDonald House or rooming-in facilities at the hospital.

Rooming-in

For various reasons, you may find the prospect of taking your baby home frightening. To lessen your fear, some hospitals offer *rooming-in,* an arrangement that allows parents to stay overnight at the hospital to care for their baby independently. Nursery staff are immediately available if needed during this time. Rooming-in lets parents see for themselves what some aspects of baby care will be like at home. Many parents feel rooming-in builds their confidence and eases the transition to home.

Timing of the rooming-in experience is important. Ideally, rooming-in should take place as close to discharge as possible. To simulate the home environment, try to have any home monitoring equipment in place during rooming-in. Rooming-in for parents who must learn about special medical equipment might be necessary for several days.

You may wish to complete your rooming-in experience a day or two before your baby's discharge date. A good night's sleep the night before discharge may help ease some of the inevitable anxiety of your baby's homecoming.

Deciding About Circumcision

Opinions vary on *circumcision* (removal of the skin covering the tip of the penis). For some, circumcision is a religious obligation, and for others, it is a personal decision. The AAP states that the health benefits of circumcision outweigh the risks of the procedure, but the benefits are not great enough to recommend universal newborn circumcision. Specific benefits include prevention of urinary tract infections, penile cancer, and transmission of some sexually transmitted infections, including HIV.

In most circumstances, the decision regarding circumcision is up to the parents to make, in the context of their religious, ethical, and cultural beliefs. If you decide that circumcision is the right choice, check with your baby's care team to discuss timing of the procedure and with your insurance carrier to see if the procedure is covered.

Preparing Yourself, Your Home, and Your Family

As your baby grows and matures, you will have a lot to do. It can be overwhelming at times. Go slowly, but don't procrastinate. Preparation gives you a chance to mobilize some of your anxious energy to make a difference in your child's future.

Preparing for an Emergency

Graduates of NICUs have a higher rate of rehospitalization than the average newborn population. Common reasons for unexpected readmission are dehydration because of vomiting or diarrhea, upper respiratory infections, or hernia complications. Know which hospital you will use, if necessary, and how to get there.

If you know your baby will come home with special medical equipment, contact public services to make sure you will receive priority help during community emergencies. The emergency medical services system (or nearest fire station) and your utility providers (water, electric, and gas) should all be aware that you have a baby with special needs in your home. Ask your baby's care team about the best way to notify these services. Also be sure to notify them when your child is no longer technology dependent or if you move.

Housecleaning

Many parents feel they must do a major cleaning to eliminate germs and dust before their baby's homecoming. This is often not necessary, and families with children and pets cannot keep up an impossible level of cleanliness.

Rely on common sense as you prepare—and maintain—your home. A thorough cleaning is enough. Harsh cleaning solutions and insecticidal sprays can leave residual odors that may irritate your baby.

Tobacco Smoke

Babies—especially those who have had or are having breathing difficulties—are at risk for a number of problems from tobacco smoke. No one should smoke in the home, around your baby, or any place where your baby spends time, such as in the car. Exposure to smoke can further damage your baby's lungs, cause ear infections and hearing problems, cause hospital admission due to bronchitis or pneumonia, and increase your baby's risk for sudden infant death syndrome (SIDS).

Pets

Pets (dogs and cats in particular) can be prepared for your baby's arrival. Bring home clothing or a blanket with your baby's scent on it before your baby is discharged. Be alert for signs of aggression or jealousy when your baby comes home, and never leave your dog or cat unsupervised near your new baby. Extra attention and discipline will solve most problems.

Thinking About Child Care

If you intend to use child care within 2 or 3 months of your baby's discharge, this is a good time to start your search. The early months at home will fly by. You'll be absorbed in your baby and your family's adjustment to this new addition. While your baby is still in the hospital, you may have more time to explore the possibilities.

Babies who will need complex care require special consideration. Quality child care for infants with special needs is often hard to find, and you may face long waiting lists. For mothers who plan to return to work quickly (maternity leave may be used up during the NICU stay), the search for child care should begin as early as possible.

Siblings

Prepare your older children for what life may be like when their baby brother or sister comes home. Plan to spend special time alone with each of your other children for a short time every day. Encourage and allow them to talk about their feelings. Most parenting books include information on helping siblings adjust to a new baby.

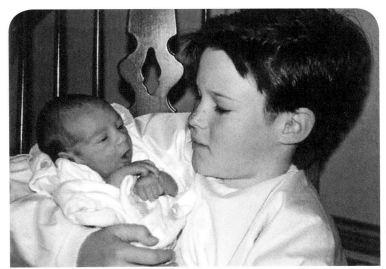

As discharge day nears, your other children may have concerns about how life will change with a new baby at home.

> We've made a lot of progress in the past few weeks. Eden is coming home! Holland won't be far behind. Both have their feeding tubes out. Holland is a wireless baby—no more tubes or monitors! Eden will come home on oxygen and a monitor. So Holland may be the breather in the family, but Eden is the eater. Today she took 50 cc while breastfeeding in 20 minutes.
>
> Billie, mother of **Holland** and **Eden**

Emotional Readiness

The days and hours before you leave the hospital are very busy and can be as stressful as the first few when you arrived. Just as you trusted the hospital staff to care for your baby, you will need to trust they know the timing of when you and the baby are ready to go home. The staff will ensure you have the skills needed and support in place and that your baby is medically ready to transition to the next phase of life—with you as competent and loving parents.

When your baby comes home, you may experience times of great stress, nights when you'll be tempted to return your baby to the hospital, and moments when you'll wonder what you ever saw in your partner. Know that these feelings will pass. Before your baby comes home, think about things you can do to help deal with your stress. Here are a few suggestions.

- Exercise; talk to a counselor, religious leader, or friend; openly express your emotions (laugh and cry); or keep a journal—but do not lock in your feelings. If you are increasingly ill, accident prone, overtired, or depressed, try something different or get help.

- You deserve an occasional break, and couples need time alone together. Have at least one support person trained to babysit all of your children. If you have home nurses, take an hour or so for yourself occasionally. Have an "at-home date" while someone else is responsible for the baby's care. Do not wait for surprise breaks in the chaos or you will be too exhausted to enjoy them.

- Pay attention to how you manage your own anxiety about your baby and his needs. It is easy to get used to being in crisis. A constant high level of worrying and watching your baby's every move is a method of trying to worry less, but it often backfires. This behavior is a sure course to burnout. Watch for changes in your baby's behavior, and develop methods of getting feedback (from a pediatrician, nurses, and friends) to help you figure things out with no panic. All in all, try to be optimistic.

- Be proud of your parenting abilities. Pat yourself on the back for getting this far. You have learned a lot about parenting and will continue to learn to trust your instincts as a parent.

- Make a list of things others could help you do. Asking for help is sometimes difficult, but this is certainly the time to do so. When people ask, "Is there anything I can do?" share your list with them. Suggestions include providing meals (freezable), shopping or running errands, doing laundry, cleaning your house, doing things with your other children, walking the dog, and doing yard work so you can rest (or play).

> After 108 days, it's really hard to believe how far our babies have come. I clearly remember the day they were born and the way they looked when we saw them for the first time. They were so beautiful and perfect but so tiny. It seemed impossible that we would ever get to this point. Now we're looking at 2 babies who will be home by the date they were expected. It's been really hard but more than worth it when I look into their sweet faces. I wouldn't trade it for anything!
>
> Billie, mother of **Holland** and **Eden**

Celebrating

Last but not least, celebrate your baby's arrival home. When your baby's health care team finally sets a discharge date, consider planning a celebration dinner with your partner before your baby is discharged. Once your baby comes home, it may be a few weeks or more before you can find much quality "couple time" in your schedules.

Discharge Day at Last!

Discharge day is exciting and frightening at the same time. Even the most prepared parents feel nervous about finally bringing their baby home.

Be prepared for delays on discharge day. You may arrive first thing in the morning, only to be told you'll have to wait for one more test, for the results of a previous test, or for a member of your baby's care team to examine your baby or write an order.

When everything is finally in place, ask for a copy of the baby's discharge summary. Some NICUs send a copy to your pediatrician. Dress your baby in the special going-home clothes you've brought with you, and ask if you may take a tour through the unit so the team can say good-bye and celebrate with you.

Some parents want to do something special for the staff. Thank-you cards, a letter to the hospital administrator expressing appreciation of the NICU and nursery staff, and letters and pictures from home are the most valuable gifts you can give the staff. They enjoy seeing the progress your baby makes.

Now you're on your way out the door with discharge instructions and bags of supplies, toys, and baby clothes. Don't forget your baby!

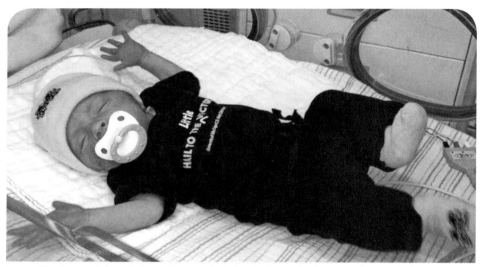

Maxwell, who was 34 weeks' gestation at admission, is dressed in his going-home clothes and ready to leave after 22 days in the NICU.

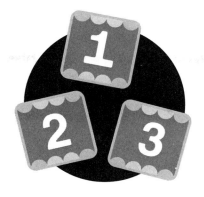

Niklas, Gabbie, & Lukas

Born at 28 weeks 4 days

In late 2006, at 28 weeks 4 days' gestation, our weekly ultrasound ended abruptly and we were escorted to a "comfy" room with flowery wallpaper to wait for the doctor. It turned out that triplet C was being deprived of the proper nutrients to survive, forcing us to make a choice to either continue with the pregnancy, knowing that triplet C would die within the next 48 hours, or have an emergency C-section. We chose the latter. Lukas was born weighing 1 pound 12 ounces, and Gabbie and Niklas were just over 2 pounds.

While waiting with Greta in the recovery room, I was told I could go visit the babies. As I was gazing at my daughter lying in the incubator, I commented to one of the nurses about the cute little baby noises she was making. I was gently told that those noises I was hearing were grunts. She was struggling to breathe and it turned out her lung had collapsed. In the course of a couple days, all 3 moved to oscillating ventilators that mechanically moved their chests up and down. Within a few hours of life, our babies had developed life-threatening respiratory distress syndrome, collapsed lungs, patent ductus arteriosus, and jaundice, and each kid suffered at least one pneumothorax (collapsed lung). Niklas developed pulmonary interstitial emphysema, and we were told it would be appropriate to say good-bye to him. He was so sick that we never actually put his crib together, as we didn't want to go through the pain of taking it apart upon his death.

About 1 week in, we received the worst news. Niklas had developed 2 brain bleeds, one in each hemisphere of his brain (an intraventricular hemorrhage)—a grade III on one side and a grade IV on the other. Grades I and II are most common, and often there are no further complications. Grades III and IV are the most serious and usually result in long-term brain injury to the infant.

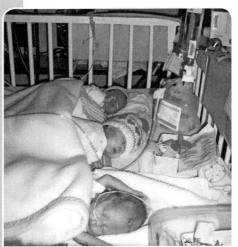

Photo of the triplets in the NICU in 2007. (The practice of co-bedding is not observed anymore.)

After a grade III or IV hemorrhage, blood clots may form, which can block the flow of cerebrospinal fluid, leading to increased fluid in the brain (hydrocephalus).

The doctors watched carefully, hoping that this situation would resolve itself. It did not. A temporary shunt was installed while we continued to see if it would resolve. It did not. A permanent shunt was then installed, which required 3 more brain surgeries to get correct. After the last surgery, we were told to expect poor eyesight, possible blindness, and likely cerebral palsy and learning disabilities. Niklas had sunset eyes after the surgery, where the irises made him look as though he were staring down—an unsettling look that we were told was permanent. After 3 months in the NICU, we brought the kids home, along with their oxygen tanks.

Today, the sunset eyes and the oxygen tanks are gone. The physical and cognitive impairments that were once certainties, never transpired. In fact, not one of our 3 kids even wears glasses. We feel very blessed that our babies were in the skilled hands of the doctors and nurses in the NICU.

Today, they are 9 years old, and we are very busy with school and after-school activities. For the most part, the triplets are average busy third graders who attend a Catholic school and enjoy learning Spanish after school. All 3 test average or above average at school.

In winter, all 3 are alpine ski enthusiasts and belong to the ski team. When ski season is over, we swim and water-ski. Last year, both boys attended sailing camp and have become good little sailors with hopes to attend the same camp again for many summers. Niklas loves taking classes and has shown an unusual talent in guitar as well as tae kwon do. Lukas is quite good at swimming and tae kwon do. Gabbie has been taking ballet classes since she was 4 years old and enjoys them to this day. Also, all 3 enjoy playing tennis.

To our pleasant surprise, all 3 have been really healthy. They don't even get common colds. I am a true believer in encouraging outdoor activities in the fresh air, sticking to strict sleep schedules, and eating a very clean diet of local or organic foods.

Jason and Greta, parents of Niklas, Gabbie, and Lukas

The triplets today.

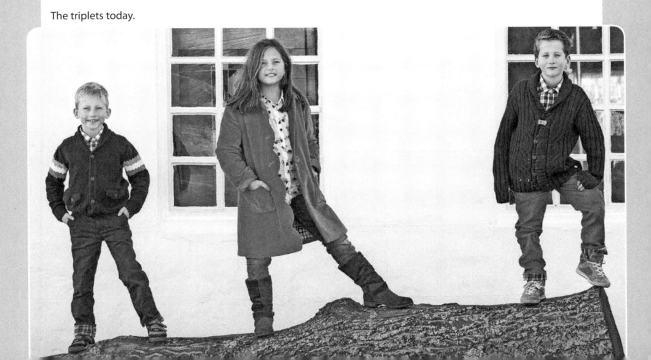

CHAPTER 9

Home at Last

"Try your hardest to not look back.
Look forward with your baby
(or babies!). Forgive yourself if you're
carrying guilt and focus on taking care
of yourself, your baby, and your
partner now."

*Kate, mother of **Lucy***

Welcome home! Your phone is ringing, your baby is crying, your children are screaming, your dog is barking, your dishes and laundry are piling up—it all seems to be too much to handle.

Bringing your baby (or babies) home can be quite overwhelming. All of the other demands of everyday life will be waiting for you, along with your new baby and the care she needs.

While your baby was in the hospital, your primary focus was on learning about her and how to meet her needs. If you were able to spend a lot of time learning to care for your baby in the neonatal intensive care unit (NICU), you have probably become quite good at the basics. If you were not able to be with your baby often, you probably got a lot of instructions before your baby was discharged. In either instance, you may find that once you get home, everything turns into chaos. Relax! This is normal for anyone with a new baby in the house, even for experienced parents. It's especially true for parents of preterm babies or others with special needs.

Parenting any baby, especially one born at risk, demands an enormous amount of adjustment. Most parents can't wait for their baby (or babies) to come home, but even the most experienced and prepared parents find the first few weeks a huge challenge.

Homecoming: You, Your Children, and Your Visitors

Even though you're relieved your baby is home, you may find that you miss the support of the hospital staff. You may feel alone and abandoned as you make the adjustment to independent parenting. For some parents, the first days at home with the baby are as stressful as their first days in the NICU.

Anxiety

You may feel highly anxious now that you have total responsibility for your baby's care and feel as though you don't remember a single thing you were taught about caring for your baby.

It may be comforting to know that you now share something with parents of healthy newborns: feelings of uncertainty and clumsiness with baby care at home. Your anxiety should diminish as you find that you are, indeed, surviving. You may do things differently than they were done in the hospital, but as long as the decisions you make keep your baby safe and thriving, you can have confidence in them.

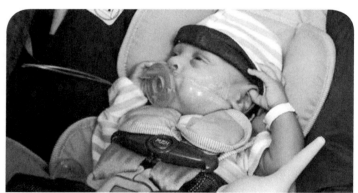

"Discharge day was one of overwhelming happiness and gratitude but also one of fear that I was leaving behind the safety net of the NICU. Thankfully, the transition went smoothly and I quickly learned how to manage the oxygen tank and apnea monitor that **Nathan** came home with and stayed on for a few months after leaving the NICU."

*Cheryl, mother of **Nathan***

Grief and Guilt

When you first started your NICU journey, you were probably told that your baby's problems were not your fault and were, in fact, outside anyone's control. Yet you may have felt guilty anyway and said to yourself, "If only I had…." Soon, though, your busy life as a NICU parent overshadowed these feelings.

Now that your baby is home, feelings of sadness and guilt may return. Parents may feel guilty when they grieve for what might have been instead of feeling grateful for the baby they have.

These feelings of grief and guilt usually pass as you gain confidence caring for your baby and adjust to your role as a parent. Support from your family, friends, and health care professionals is important to getting through this stage. Keep in mind that your own mental health goes hand in hand with your baby's healthy growth and development. Talk to someone familiar with your NICU experience; this may help with your feelings of loss of the healthy term baby you had expected.

If these feelings persist or if you continue to have upsetting memories of the NICU experience, seek help from a health care professional.

> ❝ I wish someone would have talked to me about what mental health challenges I might expect in the days, weeks, and months after we left the NICU. Post-traumatic stress, whether it reaches the level of 'disorder' or not, is common among NICU parents. That trauma for me didn't really kick in until after we went home. He'd gone into respiratory failure in my arms, so it's not surprising that I started having panic attacks. I worried, 'What if these treatments worked, but only for a short time?' When we got home, I would look at him and think, 'Well, now he's dead.' I had these thoughts many times each day and night. I was able to find a therapist who specialized in early parenthood transitions. She and the other members of my medical team were invaluable to turning my experience around and moving forward. ❞
>
> Alex, father of **Pascal**

Love and Attachment

The bonds you established with your baby during hospitalization are very real. But development of true intimacy may have been difficult because of the lack of privacy and the distractions of hospital technology. Now that your baby is home, she may suddenly seem like a little stranger. You may worry if you do not have strong feelings of love toward your baby.

Give yourself some time to get to know your baby—and to let your baby get to know you. At first, your baby will make incredible demands on your time and attention and seem to give back little. But as she grows, she will begin to respond to your efforts with quiet alertness, more frequent eye contact, and that first amazing smile. All relationships take time to grow, and with time, your love for your baby will grow.

Feeling Overwhelmed

It is not realistic to think that one person can parent a baby 24 hours a day, 7 days a week. Make a plan ahead of time so you can call on trusted friends and family to help you and care for your baby on very stressful days when you need a breather.

There is nothing bad about feeling as though you are going to "lose it" with your baby. The important thing is to recognize when you have reached your limit. Put your baby in a safe place, such as her crib, and close the door. Take a deep breath and put your support plan into action.

By following your plan, you can call a person who has agreed to help you and listen to you when you need to talk. If you do not have this kind of support, call your pediatrician's office or a parent support hotline. They can help you make a plan for keeping your baby safe while you take a few minutes to calm down.

> " Holland liked to cuddle, but at first, she fussed a bit more, and it took more trial and error to figure out what she wanted. Both girls were pretty good natured, but I must admit that I am NOT supermom! There were nights when I was so tired and cranky that my babies and I just sat and cried together! "
>
> Billie, mother of **Holland** and **Eden**

Effect on Your Older Children

The reality of the baby's homecoming is stressful for most siblings. Once the baby is home, your other children may be surprised that your attention is still focused so intensely on the baby. You can help children adjust to their new role as older brothers and sisters by suggesting activities such as a special dinner or dessert just to celebrate this new status as an older sibling. If you can, plan a small gift for each older sibling the day you bring your NICU graduate home. Involve your children's teachers, too—perhaps by sending a picture of the baby for the big brother or sister to show to classmates in a special moment.

As your children watch the baby take even more of your time, attention, and love, you may notice they seem angry at you or the baby, regress to thumb-sucking or bed-wetting, act out to get your attention, or have difficulty at school.

If older children are interested, involve them in the care of the new baby as much as possible, even though this may sometimes mean more work for you. Try not to criticize any "help" you receive, and praise a job well done. The more you can include older children in caregiving, the sooner they will adjust to the new baby's presence.

Spend some special time alone with each child, even if just for a few minutes of snuggling, reading a book, playing a game, or taking a walk together. The addition of a new baby changes your relationship with your other children, and working through this adjustment together is an important part of your growth as a parent and family.

Visitors

When your baby comes home, your friends and neighbors may assume the crisis is over and be less available for support. On the other hand, friends who were nowhere to be found during your NICU crisis may now knock on your door to see your new baby and expect to be treated as visitors.

Most health care professionals and parents of NICU graduates will tell you to limit visitors. The more people your baby is exposed to, the greater the risk of infection. Healthy visitors may be welcome, but anyone with a fever, cold, cough, open sore (such as a fever blister), or other contagious illness should not be allowed near the baby. No one should touch your baby or her belongings without washing their hands first. Good hand washing is the best prevention against illness. Most people understand when you explain that a common illness picked up from an older child or adult can develop into a serious infection for a NICU graduate.

You probably won't want to discourage all visitors because you'll need help now that your baby is home. Now more than ever, you may need to make a list of things people can do to help you, such as running errands, helping with laundry, or watching your children while you nap. Now is not the time to be super parent—ask for and accept help!

What to Expect From Your Baby

Babies are unique in the way they react to their surroundings and signal their needs. A large part of gaining confidence as a parent is feeling you are adequately meeting your baby's needs. Parenting a NICU graduate can be challenging at first, especially if your baby does not signal those needs clearly or does not act predictably.

Preterm Babies Are Different

Compared with term babies of a similar age, preterm babies are sometimes more irritable, less responsive, and less predictable. Term babies with chronic illnesses requiring NICU time may be this way too.

Try to be patient. Most babies outgrow these differences within the first year of life and grow into typical toddlers. Until that time, however, your baby may try your patience. By understanding her behavior and helping her to become more organized, you'll find it easier to get into a routine.

An important part of caring for your baby is learning what is normal and understanding how to recognize a change. A parent is often the first and best person to recognize a change in the baby's general condition, including positive changes and potential concerns or changes in behavior, which should be brought to the doctor's attention.

Corrected Age

If your baby was born early, she has 2 important days to mark on the calendar. The day your baby was born is her official date of birth, but her estimated due date is also an important day. When you measure your baby's development—that is, when you look at what is "normal" for your baby's age—consider both of those dates. By looking at the difference between them, you can adjust her calendar age to account for her prematurity and calculate her corrected age. During the first 2 years, using her corrected age will give you a better idea when she should reach common developmental goals.

Calculating corrected age isn't difficult. Begin with your baby's actual age in weeks (number of weeks since the date of birth) and then subtract the number of weeks your baby was preterm. This is your baby's corrected age. A term pregnancy is 40 weeks' gestation. To determine the number of weeks' preterm your baby was at birth, subtract her gestational age at birth from 40. For example, if your baby was born at 32 weeks' gestation, she was 8 weeks (2 months) preterm. If she is now 4 months old (16 weeks since birth), her corrected age is 2 months.

Actual age in weeks minus	Weeks preterm	=	Corrected age
16 weeks since birth –	8 weeks	=	8 weeks (2 months)

In this case, even if your baby is 4 months old, you should expect her to have the developmental skills of a 2-month-old term baby. It would be unrealistic to expect your baby to be ready to roll from her stomach to her back—a skill that often develops in term babies around the age of 4 months. Your baby may just be beginning to hold her head up and smile, which is developmentally normal for a term baby of 2 months and, therefore, for a preterm baby whose corrected age is 2 months.

Parents are often frustrated by well-meaning family and friends who express concerns about their baby's development. People may think your baby is delayed for a 4-month-old, for example, when, in fact, she is on target for a baby with a corrected age of 2 months.

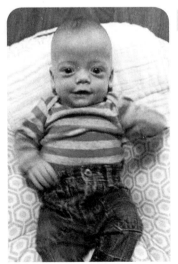

Sleep Patterns

Don't expect your preterm baby to sleep through the night for many months. Unlike a term baby, who might sleep a full 6 to 8 hours at night by 4 months of age, your baby may not sleep through the night until 6 to 8 months or later. Until your baby develops a regular sleep cycle, help her to fall asleep at night by separating daytime and nighttime activities. Talk and play with your baby during daytime awake periods. Keep night feedings calm and quiet. This will help your baby learn the difference between day and night and may help you get much-needed sleep. Try to put your baby to bed when she is drowsy but still awake. Becoming used to falling asleep on her own may help her fall back to sleep if she wakes up during the night.

"We were lucky. **Auggie** was always smiling and so happy."

*Robyn, mother of **Auggie***

Babies vary in how easily they settle down to sleep. Follow the same steps each time you put your baby down to sleep to help her learn a personal going-to-sleep routine.

Fussing and Crying

Although your baby will sleep up to 16 hours a day at first, her actual sleep times may be short. She may awaken and fuss every 2 to 3 hours until 3 to 4 months' corrected age. She may wake up and fuss even if she is not hungry.

Try holding her with her arms and legs tucked closely to her body and rocking her while you stand or sit in a rocking chair. Some babies prefer a gentle up-and-down motion over side-to-side movement. Your baby may prefer a walk in your arms or in a stroller or carriage. Some babies find a rocking swing comforting, but only use a swing if your baby passed the car safety seat test, has no respiratory problems in a sitting position, and is big enough to sit safely. Other babies like singing and hearing music or "white noise" from a vacuum cleaner, clothes dryer, or fan. A warm bath may be calming. Still others enjoy being gently patted, massaged, held skin-to-skin on your chest, swaddled snugly (but not too tightly), or going for a ride in the car. Many babies find sucking on their hand or a pacifier comforting. Try one thing at a time and you'll learn what works best.

If your baby is unusually fussy or will not settle, check to see if something could be causing pain (for example, the sharp edge of a clothing tag, a hair wrapped tightly around a finger or toe, an eyelash in your baby's eye) and check to see if your baby is feverish or for other signs of illness.

Many babies go through a fussy or "colicky" period that begins anywhere from 2 to 4 weeks' corrected age, peaks around 6 weeks' corrected age, and usually resolves by 3 months' corrected age but can last until 6 months' corrected age. For some babies, this fussy period occurs at the same time every day (usually late afternoon or early evening). Fussy periods also happen when your baby is eating while becoming more alert and aware of her environment. In other words, your baby becomes overwhelmed by the end of the day and needs a good cry to help her relax! But getting her to calm down may be a challenge.

During your baby's first months at home, you'll be learning what she likes and doesn't like. The most frustrating thing for parents is that the same comfort measure doesn't work every time—and may not work 2 times in a row. When you find something that works, stick with it until it doesn't work any longer. Babies like consistency and rituals, especially as they get older.

Consider placing your baby in a front pouch and "wearing" her around the house. If you're doing active chores or cooking, be sure to keep safety in mind. This technique may make your baby cry less and enhance her learning. Check with your baby's doctor before using a baby pack or pouch—sometimes, NICU graduates do not have enough muscle strength to keep their airways open in an unsupported position.

Some parents worry about spoiling their baby with too much holding. Don't worry. Experts agree that holding a baby meets her basic need to feel safe. In fact, babies who are picked up as soon as they begin to cry tend to cry less often and for shorter periods than do babies whose parents don't respond quickly.

This doesn't mean you have to pick your baby up with every peep you hear. As your baby grows, let her learn about and explore personal ways to self-comfort. She will discover that sucking her fist, holding her blanket, or clasping her hands together will help her feel better for a few moments.

How long to let your baby cry remains controversial. If your baby has special needs and turns blue with crying, your choice is clear and you will need to respond quickly. If your baby is healthy, you can make a parenting choice. Some baby care experts feel you should never let your baby cry it out alone. They recommend a quick response to your baby's cry to meet the need for security and to let your baby know she is important.

Some babies seem to need to cry themselves to sleep and will not be comforted no matter what you try. If your baby is very fussy every day, make a plan for someone to give you a break, even if only for an hour or so. You will need a break so you can return to your baby feeling more relaxed and calm.

Whether you decide to respond to your baby's cry immediately or wait a moment, the important thing is to do what you feel is right. Trust your instincts. Try a combination of approaches before you decide which one is right for you and your baby.

Concerns About Feeding

Now that your baby is home, you'll be making more independent decisions about when and how much your baby eats. Some parents discover things they didn't learn about their baby's eating habits while the baby was in the hospital and wonder if they are "doing it right" at home.

Breastfeeding your preterm baby or baby with special needs at home can be challenging. You can use the resources available in your community, including your pediatrician, a lactation consultant, or a support group, to help you stay inspired and confident in your abilities.

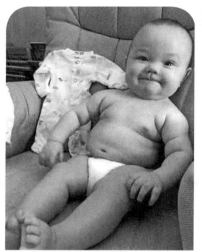

Lucy shows how much she's grown by posing next to her preemie outfit.

Helping Your Baby Eat Well

A calm place to eat is important for all babies but especially for those who become stressed from too much stimulation. Watch your baby's cues during the feeding. Does she yawn, sneeze, hiccup, get frantic, or lose interest and fall asleep in the middle of feeding? Talking into your baby's face or feeding your baby near the television may be too much for your baby to handle.

Tips for a Successful Feeding Experience

- If you are bottle-feeding formula, prepare the formula in advance. If you warm the formula, do not use a microwave oven because the bottle may be heated unevenly and you could scald your baby's mouth. Place the bottle in hot water or a bottle warmer, instead, and check the temperature of the milk against your wrist to make sure it is lukewarm.
- Minimize distractions in the room. Dim the lights a bit and turn down the television or radio.
- Support your baby's head, neck, and hips, flexing the hips slightly.
- To help your baby anticipate the feeding, place your finger or a few drops of breast milk or formula on her lips.
- If necessary, gently support your baby's jaw with your finger to keep the milk in her mouth.
- Find the right bottle and nipple for your baby. You should know this before hospital discharge.
- Watch for signs of stress, and give her a break when necessary.
- Give your baby quiet time to recover after the feeding is over.
- Never put your baby to sleep with a bottle propped in her mouth or allow her to sleep with a bottle. She could easily choke, and bottle propping leads to baby tooth decay and, possibly, ear infections.

How Much and How Often to Feed

Before your baby's discharge, the NICU team should have explained her feeding plan and provided you with written instructions. These instructions probably included how much and how often to feed her. Special preterm discharge formulas designed specifically for growing preterm babies are sometimes continued after discharge to help with weight gain during the transition to home. Some babies need a specific feeding schedule after discharge. Your pediatrician may adjust that schedule only after weighing and examining your baby in the office. Other babies may be able to feed *on demand* or *ad lib,* meaning the baby determines how much and how often to eat, according to her feeding readiness cues.

If you'll be feeding your baby on demand at home, you should begin to feed her this way before discharge. This will give you an opportunity to learn your baby's cues that signal readiness to eat. If your baby's feeding cues are not fully mature at the time of discharge, the recommendation may be to feed your baby on demand but offer a feeding at least every 3 to 4 hours with a minimum of 6 to 8 feedings per day.

Your NICU team may suggest you use a combination of feeding methods for your growing preterm baby at the time of discharge. You may be asked to breastfeed a certain number of feedings each day, use an alternate method for the other feedings, and gradually increase the frequency of breastfeeding while your baby's weight gain is monitored. Between breastfeeding, you can provide either breast milk or formula by using a bottle or supplemental nursing device, finger feeding, or cup feeding. Whenever you are supplementing your baby's feedings (with breast milk or formula), it is important for the mother to continue to pump milk after every feeding to maintain or build the mother's milk supply. Supplementation without pumping allows your baby to be fed but does not provide the stimulation necessary to continue making milk.

As your baby grows, so should her appetite. If your baby takes less than what she needs at a feeding, she may wake up earlier or take more at the next feeding. If she takes in too much or eats too quickly, she may spit up. Once she is able to take in more at each feeding, the time between feedings may lengthen. It's particularly nice when your baby starts lengthening the time between feedings at night, letting you get more sleep.

Clearly, feeding schedules need to be individualized depending on your baby's ability and weight gain. Visits with your pediatrician, home health nurse, or a lactation specialist during the first week or two after discharge (and for as long as necessary after that) can help to resolve any ongoing feeding issues.

> **❝** Eden is home! She weighed 5 pounds 1.5 ounces when she left the NICU and 5 pounds 5.5 ounces today at her pediatrician appointment. I think we're growing her good! We're continuing to breastfeed twice a day until she gets bigger and we can move toward full time (that's my goal!). **❞**
>
> Billie, mother of **Holland** and **Eden**

How Long to Feed

Feeding length varies, depending on how frequently your baby wants to eat and how easily she tires while feeding. Breastfed babies may begin nursing only a few minutes on each side and may require more frequent feedings. You should hear sucking and swallowing, along with some pauses. Gradually, your baby may work up to nursing 20 minutes or more on each side. The usual length of time it takes a breastfed baby to complete a feeding is about 20 minutes. Healthy preterm newborns who do not have any health issues, especially respiratory problems, may want to nurse for up to 40 minutes. As long as your baby does not seem exhausted, seems content after feeding, and is gaining weight (weight checks may need to be done at home or in the doctor's office), there's no reason to limit feeding time. In fact, your baby may become frustrated if you end the feeding too soon. Babies nurse not only to satisfy hunger but also to satisfy their need for sucking, security, and comfort. Falling asleep or ceasing to suck are the usual indicators that a feeding is over.

In general, a feeding by bottle finishes more quickly than a feeding at the breast, but this also depends on how vigorously the baby sucks and swallows and how often the baby needs to take a break. Some NICU graduates feed from the bottle until they become tired (you will recognize these signs from learning to feed your baby in the NICU) and finish the feeding by gavage (a feeding tube). Gradually, your baby will gain strength and you'll notice improvement in her feeding abilities, so there is no need to push her. Your baby will have more difficulty gaining weight if she uses all of her calories to get through long, perhaps stressful, feeding periods.

Weight Gain

As you settle into a feeding routine, you may wonder whether your baby is gaining enough weight. Optimal weight gain is approximately 15 g (½ oz) per day before your baby's due date and 20 to 30 g (a little more than ½ to 1 oz) per day for the first 6 months. You're aiming for a weight gain of 1 pound per month. Your baby's pediatrician will plot measurements of weight, length, and head circumference on her growth chart. Your pediatrician may recommend weekly weight checks at the office or at home by a visiting nurse to check for adequate weight gain for the first few weeks (or longer) after discharge.

Feeding Problems

Some babies are more difficult to feed than others. Even though you practiced feeding your baby in the hospital, some problems may persist after your baby comes home.

A bottle-feeding baby who gulps rapidly and then spits everything up may need a nipple that delivers the milk more slowly. You might need to try a few different types of standard bottle nipples before you find the one that works best. You may need to regulate the length of time the nipple is in your baby's mouth as well. Frequent burping and feeding the baby in a more upright position may also help prevent spitting up.

If your baby tends to hold her breath or gulp her food, your NICU nurse probably helped you watch her breathing pattern and color during feedings. Preterm babies frequently have trouble coordinating sucking, swallowing and breathing during a feeding. If you notice breath holding or a color change (to pale, dusky, or blue) at any time during a feeding, take the nipple out of your baby's mouth. Try gentle stimulation—rubbing or patting your baby's back, for example— to remind her to breathe. The rubbing or patting may also bring up a burp. As preterm babies mature, their coordination improves. If this is a new behavior for your baby or if she is having more frequent breathing trouble during feedings, call your pediatrician at once.

If you have difficulty feeding your baby after discharge, contact your pediatrician. Frequently, all you need is some advice and reassurance from a health care professional who is familiar with your baby's eating habits.

A Feeding Log

Whether your baby is breastfeeding or bottle-feeding, you may want to keep a log of each feeding for the first few weeks at home. Keeping a log is a simple and valuable way to work in partnership with your baby's pediatrician. Use a notebook to document

- Feeding times

- Time at breast or amount per bottle

- Any feeding difficulties

- Wet and dirty diapers

- Special comments (for example, is your baby satisfied after a feeding or does she cry a lot; does your baby fall asleep in the middle of the feeding; does your baby need to be awakened for feedings?)

Bring this information with you when you take your baby to your pediatrician. Appointments at the pediatrician's office are often only 15 minutes long, giving you little time to organize your questions. If you come prepared with your written questions and feeding log, you will be able to make the most of your office visit. Once your baby has established a consistent pattern of feeding and gaining weight for you at home, you can comfortably retire your feeding log as part of your baby book.

> Lucy could not breastfeed when she was discharged and it took her another 2 months after we came home to get it. At 17 months old, it is definitely her favorite pastime. This is so hard to believe after what a struggle it once was for her.
>
> Kate, mother of Lucy

Other Common Homecoming Concerns

It may have seemed like an eternity until you were able to take your baby home. Now, at last, you have control over your baby and your family life—or do you? The normal elements of baby care may not be so routine for you. The first few days, weeks, and even months at home may, in fact, be unsettling. Here are some common concerns, with the goal of helping you to organize your family life once again.

Sudden Infant Death Syndrome (SIDS)

Many parents worry about their baby's chances of death from sudden infant death syndrome (SIDS), sometimes called *crib death*. Sudden infant death syndrome is the sudden, unexplained death of a baby younger than 1 year that doesn't have a known cause even after a complete investigation. Babies can also die while in a sleep environment from accidental causes, such as accidental suffocation or strangulation, or from ill-defined causes.

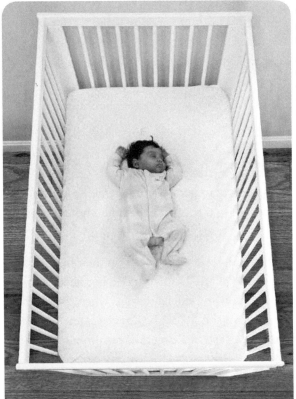

Your baby should sleep on her back on a firm mattress covered with a fitted sheet and with no fluffy bedding or objects around her.

Image courtesy of the Safe to Sleep® campaign, for educational purposes only; Eunice Kennedy Shriver National Institute of Child Health and Human Development, http://safetosleep.nichd.nih.gov; Safe to Sleep® is a registered trademark of the US Department of Health and Human Services.

Reducing the Risk of SIDS and Sleep-Related Deaths

There are a number of things you can do to create a safe sleep environment for your baby.

- Always place your baby to sleep on her back, for naps and at night.

- Place your baby on a firm mattress covered with a fitted sheet. There should be no other bedding or soft objects in the sleep area.

- If your baby falls asleep in a car safety seat, stroller, swing, or infant carrier, she should be moved to a firm sleep surface as soon as possible.

- Avoid sleep positioning devices sold to parents with the claim that they position babies for safe sleep or that are inconsistent with safe sleep recommendations.

- Make sure nothing is covering your baby's head.

- Your baby should sleep in your room, close to your bed, but on a separate surface designed for babies. Share your room, but don't share your bed. Never place your baby for sleep on a couch, sofa, or armchair.

- Breastfeed your baby.

- Offer a dry pacifier at sleep time throughout the first year of life. If your baby doesn't want it or if it falls out of her mouth, do not force it or prop the pacifier in place. Do not hang the pacifier around your baby's neck, and do not attach the pacifier to your baby's clothing while sleeping.

- Don't smoke or allow smoking around your baby. Talk with your doctor about getting help to quit smoking.

- Don't use fluffy or loose bedding, pillows, beanbags, or water beds.

- Don't overdress or over-bundle your baby and don't overheat your baby's room. Your baby should be lightly clothed or in a sleep sack, and the bedroom temperature should feel comfortable to a lightly clothed adult. Your baby should not feel hot to the touch and should not be sweating.

- Do not use home cardiorespiratory monitors. They do not reduce the risk of SIDS.

All babies, including preterm and low birth weight babies, should be placed on their back to sleep. You may have seen your baby nested on her stomach in the NICU surrounded by rolled blankets. This was done at an earlier time in your baby's life for specific medical reasons when the baby was on continuous heart rate and respiratory monitoring. This should not be done at home. A small number of babies with special medical conditions may sleep in a different position, but your baby's pediatrician will discuss this with you.

For additional information about how to decrease the risk of SIDS and sleep-related deaths, visit the official AAP Web site for parents, **www.HealthyChildren.org**.

Concerns About Back Sleeping

Most new parents are aware of the recommendations for positioning babies on their back to sleep. Your parents or grandparents, however, raised "tummy sleepers" and may have the following concerns about back sleeping:

- **Choking:** The most common fear about the back-sleeping position is that the baby will spit up and choke while asleep. Healthy NICU graduates are able to turn their heads or protect their airways if they spit up.

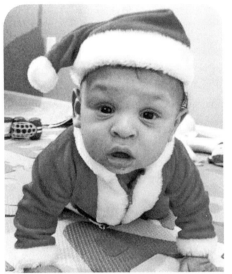

Nathan (Santa's helper) built some muscle during "tummy time" and can now lift his chest off the floor with his arms.

- **Flat head:** Technically called *positional plagiocephaly,* your baby's head may be flat in the back and narrow on the sides. The head usually rounds out as the baby matures, holds her head up independently, and spends less time on her back. Encourage plenty of supervised tummy time when your baby is awake, and avoid placing your baby in car safety seat carriers or "bouncers" for long lengths of time. Frequently change the position your baby faces in the crib or change the crib to the other side of the room so she is not always lying on the same side of her head. If plagiocephaly occurs despite these preventive measures, talk with your pediatrician about possible treatment options.

- **Delayed development:** Allowing the baby plenty of supervised time on her tummy while she's awake will build the necessary neck and shoulder muscles she needs to roll over.

Family Bed: Not Recommended

Your friends may have shared their bed with their newborn or young children. As research emerged on SIDS risk factors, the AAP determined that the safest place for your baby to sleep is in the room where you sleep but not in your bed and not in the same bed with another baby.

Placing your baby's crib or bassinet near your bed (within arm's reach) will make breastfeeding easier and allow you to better watch over your baby. This is especially true for parents of babies who require frequent nighttime feedings or who have special needs, such as medical treatments around the clock. Sudden infant death syndrome prevention studies recommend that babies should sleep in their parents' room for the first 6 months of life.

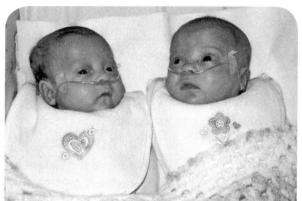

"Our lives now are busy, busy, busy, and without much sleep. The babies never sleep for more than a 3-hour stretch. It was OK at first, but that kind of sleeping schedule really catches up with you. When they wake up at 4:00 am, it takes over an hour for us to warm bottles, feed and burp, pump, and clean up, so I don't get back to sleep until around 5:15 am, only to wake up again around 7:45 am. I guess that's the life of a mommy. On top of all that normal baby stuff, we are also dealing with 2 to 3 doctor appointments a week, medicine schedules, and all kinds of equipment and alarms."

Billie, mother of **Holland** *and* **Eden**

Your baby should sleep in her own safety-approved crib or bassinet, on a firm mattress, with a fitted sheet. Do not use crib bumpers. Never put your baby in your bed or on a chair, sofa, or water bed to sleep. It is safer to use sleep clothing or sleep sacks instead of a blanket to avoid overheating. Blankets should not be used for "nesting" or to provide boundaries for your baby. Finally, it is important to keep all pillows, quilts, comforters, sheepskin, and stuffed toys out of your baby's crib. They can cover your baby's face and suffocate her—even if she is positioned on her back.

Bathing

As long as you keep your baby's face, neck, skinfolds, and diaper area clean, you don't have to bathe her every day. A sponge bath will be fine until your baby can tolerate a tub bath without much stress. Some parents get into the tub with their baby to hold and snuggle as they wash. This provides skin-to-skin contact for you and your baby. Hold your baby securely and be sure the bathwater isn't too hot for your baby.

There are only 2 rules for tub bathing your baby: Don't let your baby get cold, and keep your baby safe.

Never leave your baby unattended in the tub. If the doorbell rings and you must answer it, wrap the baby in a towel and take her with you. If you must reach for something or turn away, keep one hand securely on your baby.

Bathe your baby in the warmest area of the house—preferably one free from drafts. You'll need only a few inches of water that feels comfortably warm to your wrist or elbow. Your baby will be slippery when wet; try placing a soft towel or preformed sponge insert in the bottom of the tub. Use a mild soap to wash your baby's body. No soap is needed on your baby's face. Most pediatricians advise against the routine use of lotions and powders.

If your son was circumcised, you were probably instructed not to tub bathe him until the circumcision is healed. If you chose not to have your baby circumcised, you simply need to wash the penis at bath time. Don't try to pull back the foreskin. It will naturally separate from the penis over several years, and as your son grows, you'll teach him to wash carefully as part of his daily routine.

Keeping Your Baby Warm Enough

Before discharge, you learned how to take your baby's temperature. Unless you've been instructed to check your baby's temperature routinely, you'll probably take it only when you suspect illness. But how can you tell if your baby is maintaining a comfortable body temperature?

It's not necessary (and not recommended) to turn your heat up to a sweltering level to keep your baby warm. A normal household temperature that is comfortable for an adult in light clothing is recommended and is fine for most babies. If you have special concerns, ask your baby's doctor for advice.

Dress your baby in the same clothing or one more layer than you would wear to feel comforable. If you're comfortable in a T-shirt and shorts, for example, your baby may need a footed jumper suit. On a cooler day, when you need a shirt and a pullover sweater, dress your baby in a jumper suit and a sweater. Avoid the temptation to overdress (and overheat) your baby. A baby who is dressed too warmly may fuss, turn red, and possibly sweat. The temperature of a baby's hands or feet may not be reliable, but if her tummy feels cool, add a layer of clothing.

Outings

Use common sense when deciding about outings. There's probably no reason why your baby can't sit outside in the shade with you on a nice spring day or go with you to a friend's house

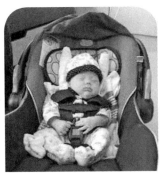

for lunch. Avoid any exposure to direct sunlight in the spring and summer months. Even a short period in direct sun can result in sunburn at this stage.

Most health care professionals suggest limiting your baby's exposures for the first 1 to 2 months at home. Fall and winter months are especially bad for cold and flu viruses that could put your NICU graduate back into the hospital, but contagious viruses are even present in the spring and summer months. If you do take

Lucy is secured safely in her car seat for one of her first outings.

your baby out, avoid crowded places and limit the number of people who have direct contact with your baby. Anyone who touches your baby must first wash their hands or use an alcohol hand sanitizer.

> 66 I learned a lot from the nurses—to change and then feed instead of the other way around, the amazingness of swaddling, the miracle of diaper rash cream. Even Pascal's struggle with the car seat test taught me a lot about car seat safety and getting a baby positioned well. I wouldn't be the dad I am without the NICU. 99
>
> Alex, father of **Pascal**

Babysitters and Child Care

Because you may limit your baby's outings and visitors for the first few months at home, you may be wondering what to do when you need to go out. Anyone who watches your baby while you are away, whether that person is a babysitter, grandparent, or other relative or friend, should know how to manage your baby's needs and understand safe sleep positioning. Ideally, all of your babysitters should complete an infant cardiopulmonary resuscitation (CPR) course. Some hospitals offer CPR courses for NICU parents and caregivers. If your hospital does not offer a CPR course, consider using the American Heart Association (AHA)/AAP *Infant CPR Anytime* program. This is a self-directed personal training kit that allows anyone to learn how to perform infant CPR in about 20 minutes.

Check your babysitter's references and ask about previous child care experience. If you are using out-of-home child care, it is important to look carefully at the child care facilities in your area and consider some important points.

Choosing Child Care for Your Baby

- Choose a state-certified/licensed child care facility and make sure that every child care worker is certified in infant and child CPR according to AHA guidelines.

- Check with consumer groups and your state's licensing authority to make sure there have been no unresolved complaints or health violations made against the facility.

- Ask the director about infant sleep position practices and if the facility has ever cared for infants who were born preterm or have special needs.

- Ask about visitation policies. You should be allowed to visit the facility anytime so you can really see staff interact with infants and toddlers. Some facilities have special webcams so you can view your baby at any time during the day while you are at work.

- Pay particular attention to child care workers' hand-washing practices and whether or not they use gloves when changing diapers. Are there sinks and soap near the cribs?

- Look at the storage area for breast milk and formula. Are bottles clearly labeled? What precautions are taken to decrease the risk of feeding a baby the wrong formula or someone else's breast milk?

- What is the caregiver to baby ratio? The lower the ratio, the better it is for your preterm baby or NICU graduate. Keep in mind that child care centers that foster developmental care and offer low worker to baby ratios tend to be more expensive and in demand and have longer waiting lists.

- For more information on choosing a quality child care center, visit the official AAP Web site for parents, **www.HealthyChildren.org**.

Secondhand and Thirdhand Smoke

Secondhand smoke is exhaled smoke and the smoke that comes from the tip of a burning cigarette, pipe, or cigar. It contains thousands of dangerous chemicals, with more than 50 of them known to cause cancer. Thirdhand smoke is the contamination that remains after the cigarette is put out. Thirdhand smoke is found on the clothing and furniture of a smoker and in the car where a smoker uses tobacco. Anytime your baby is near someone who has been smoking, she is exposed to these chemicals (as are you).

Babies and children exposed to smoke from these sources have a higher risk of serious health problems, including SIDS, ear infections, respiratory problems, allergies, and asthma.

It is important to create a smoke-free environment for you, your baby, and your family. Ban smoking in your house (put a sign on your front door as a reminder if necessary) and anyplace where your baby spends time. If your baby's caregivers smoke, they should change or cover their clothing after smoking and before they come near your baby. Avoid places that are not smoke-free and be aware that secondhand and thirdhand smoke are damaging to your baby's health and development.

Protecting Your Baby From Illness

Many parents feel like paramedics in training throughout their children's lives. The first fever, the first rash, the first fall off the tricycle all present new experiences in assessment and treatment. It's too bad that we can't wave a magic wand and protect our babies from illness and injury once they're home. The possibility of illness is especially frightening for parents of preterm babies or babies with special needs, who have already had to overcome many obstacles just to get home. Most parents learn, through experience, the difference between serious and minor problems.

Strategies to Avoid Illness

Good hand washing is the best way to prevent the spread of infection. Always wash your hands (and your other children's hands) when you arrive home from work, child care, or school. Wash your hands after you change a diaper and, of course, after you use the bathroom.

You know to limit visitors soon after your baby's arrival home and to ask friends or family with illnesses not to visit. But what if you or someone in your household gets sick? How do you keep your baby from getting the illness?

If possible, someone who is not sick should do most of the baby care if you are sick. Keeping ill siblings away from their baby sister or brother can be difficult; it may be easier to keep the baby away from them. A careful explanation may help if the ill child is old enough to understand that your baby could easily catch his or her illness.

Good hand washing is extra important if you or someone in your family has a cold, the flu, a fever, or a stomach or diarrheal illness. Wash your hands before you pick up your baby, after

> ❝ Holland was in the hospital with pneumonia, and then sick again with a cold and ear infection a mere 3 weeks later! We went back on lockdown! No one visited unless they had been symptom-free for at least 48 hours, and anyone who approached our babies had to wash their hands! It's one thing when you have a normal kid who gets a cold and gets over it. It's a whole different scene when you have to worry that your kid is going to end up in the hospital because she can't breathe with every little cold she gets. ❞
>
> Billie, mother of **Holland** and **Eden**

you blow your nose, after you sneeze or cough into your hands, and before breastfeeding or preparing a bottle. Do not allow sick people to kiss or get too close to the baby's face, especially if they have a respiratory illness or cold sore (fever blister).

Keep everyone in your family and those who have frequent contact with your baby up-to-date on their immunizations. This is an easy step to protect your baby from preventable, and often devastating, diseases (see Chapter 8).

Working With Your Baby's Pediatrician

If your baby is a healthy NICU graduate with few or no complications, most illnesses will run their course without problems. If your baby was very preterm or has ongoing health problems at home, illness may represent a greater threat.

Ask your pediatrician when you should call about a suspected illness. If your baby has special health needs, talk about what kind of problems can be expected and which ones can be managed at home. Seeing your pediatrician on a regular basis for the first few months gives you the opportunity to get answers to all of your what-if questions and may save anxious visits to the emergency department in the middle of the night.

Knowing how much care and monitoring your baby required in the NICU, you may be concerned you won't be able to tell when your baby is getting sick at home. All babies get sick, but not every illness is life-threatening. You'll quickly learn your baby's normal behavior and will be the best person to determine when something is not right. Trust your instincts.

Signs of Illness to Report to Your Pediatrician

Some signs of illness include

- Fever (a temperature higher than 100.4°F [38°C] rectally). The rectal route is recommended until your baby reaches at least 6 months of age (or until your pediatrician gives you the go-ahead to use a different route).
- Difficulty breathing (faster and harder, using more effort or grunting, noisy breathing).
- Lack of interest in eating or not feeding as well as usual.
- Vomiting most or all feedings (different from the usual amount if your baby frequently spits up food) or vomit that is dark green or bloody.
- Watery stools that soak into the diaper.
- More crying and irritability than usual (calming and comforting don't work as usual) or refusal to sleep.
- Change in color: pale, bluish, or blotchy (*mottled*) appearance.
- Behavior that is "just not right"; for example, less activity than usual, more sleeping, more difficulty waking.

It's important to know when your baby is not acting like herself, but you aren't expected to be the doctor. When you have concerns about illness, call your pediatrician. Most offices expect calls from concerned parents and have experienced staff ready to help you. If you call after hours and get the answering service, be sure to include any special circumstances with your baby (for example, say that your baby is a NICU graduate on home oxygen) in case a pediatrician who is not familiar with your baby's history receives the message. That will help ensure a speedy response to your call.

Be ready to supply the following information:

- Why you think your baby is ill

- The baby's temperature and how you took the temperature (A rectal temperature is most accurate in a baby.)

- Current medications, any new medications or recently discontinued medications, and recent immunizations

Taking Your Baby's Temperature

The most reliable way to determine a baby's body temperature is to take your baby's rectal temperature with a digital electronic thermometer.

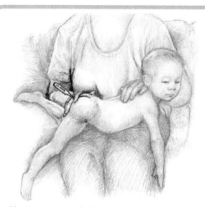

The recommended position for your baby is lying on her tummy over your legs or on a firm surface, such as a changing table. This lets you control your baby's movements and prevents her from rolling onto the thermometer, which could cause an injury.

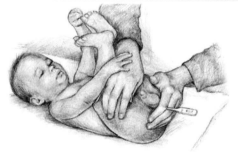

After your baby is home, if you suspect your baby has a fever, your baby's doctor will probably ask you to take a rectal temperature.

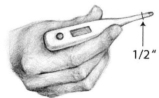

1/2"

The thermometer should be inserted ½ inch into the rectum. Never force a rectal thermometer.

Taking a rectal temperature.

Giving Medications: Missed or Vomited Doses

If your baby must take medications at home, you need to know the name, purpose, dose (how much), possible side effects, when to give each medication to your baby, and how to give each medication to your baby. You should have received this information before discharge. Tack this information to your bulletin board or tape it to your refrigerator door for handy reference and keep a copy with you.

Give all medications as directed by your baby's doctor. Most medications work best when a steady level is maintained in the body. If you forget a dose or your baby vomits shortly after you give a dose, wait until the next regularly scheduled time to give another dose. Missing one dose of a medication is usually not a problem. Check with your baby's doctor or nurse before trying to give another dose before the next scheduled time because *some medications should not be repeated under any circumstances.* Never try to make up for a missed or vomited dose by doubling or increasing the next dose.

Call your doctor if your baby misses or vomits 2 regularly scheduled doses or if she begins to vomit more feedings than usual. Depending on the medication your baby is taking, your doctor may want to check the level of medication in your baby's blood. Also notify your doctor if your baby experiences any of the potential adverse side effects associated with a medication.

Basic Rules for Medications

Don't forget these basic rules about medications.

- Keep all medications out of the reach of children.
- Use the dosing device (syringe or medicine cup) that came with the medicine. Do not use your regular silverware or household measuring spoons to estimate a dosage.
- Do not give your baby nonprescription medicines without asking your baby's doctor, especially cough and cold syrups, which may have side effects that are dangerous to your baby.
- Fever medicine, such as acetaminophen (for example, Tylenol) or ibuprofen (for example, Advil), should not be given to babies younger than 3 months without asking a health care professional first. Never give your baby aspirin.
- Do not use old prescription medicines or another child's prescription medicine.
- Find out how to store the medication; for example, some medicines require refrigeration.
- Always use child-resistant safety caps.
- Do not give medication in the dark. Be sure you have enough light to read the label, measure the dose, and see that your baby actually took the medication.

On Your Own

Your baby's homecoming is a big event. Homecoming is also an adjustment—a time of shifting values, expectations, and priorities. Parents of NICU graduates have all of the concerns of parents of healthy term babies, and then some. Don't isolate yourself and try to handle everything alone. Find people who can and will support you. Take a moment to appreciate those who have helped you get to this point, and be proud of all you have learned about caring for your new baby.

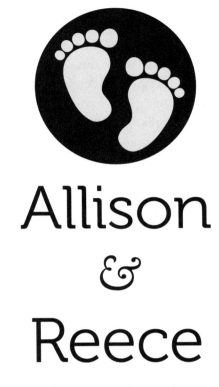

Allison
&
Reece

Born at 33 weeks
· · · · · · · · · · · · · ·

Born just shy of 33 weeks, Allison and Reece were 3 pounds 7 ounces and 4 pounds 8 ounces, respectively. Allison's water broke at 28 weeks, but with close monitoring, doctors were able to help delay their births for 5 weeks. While this was a very scary and uncertain time for us and their siblings, it was priceless for their development. An infection eventually called for an emergency C-section. They spent almost a month in the NICU, first receiving respiratory care and treatment for jaundice, and then focusing on growing and learning to eat. The circumstances resulted in a disappointing breastfeeding experience. We also faced the challenges of different NICU release dates, but in the end, the result of 2 healthy, happy children is priceless!

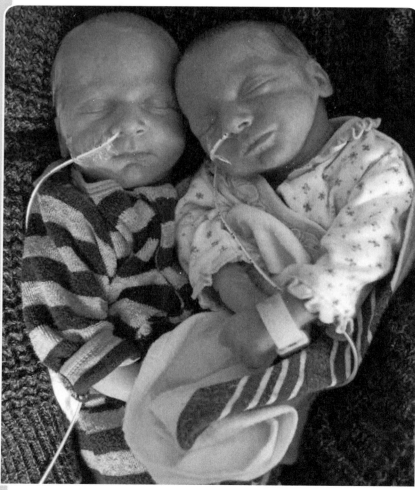

Reese and Allison, at 15 days old.

From the beginning, Allison and Reece have been distinctly different individuals. Allison, with big, expressive eyes, always needed more attention as a baby, while Reece was more easygoing and a better sleeper. As they became toddlers, Allison was the alpha twin who showed more independence and mothered Reece, while Reece was happy to follow along. He also had some speech delays but is on track now. While they fight, as all siblings do, they play well together using their amazing imaginations, and their twin bond is unquestionable. Allison creates elaborate scenes with her dolls and ponies, while Reece prefers things with wheels and learning facts about "our world." Together, they craft endlessly and love to be outside.

Gudrun, mother of Allison and Reece

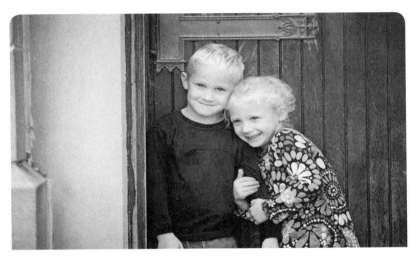

Reese and Allison, today.

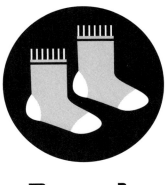

Jack

Born at 29 weeks

· ·

&

Henry

Born at 31 weeks

· ·

Jack

- Born in 2009

- Weight: 2 pounds 11 ounces

- Length: 15 inches

- Gestational age: 29 weeks

- NICU stay: 56 days

Jack had a number of complications when he was born, mainly breathing issues. He was on and off a ventilator for the first few days. He did go home on oxygen and a monitor. He also had monthly follow-ups with the developmental clinic to monitor his progress.

Today, Jack is a happy, healthy 6-year-old. He has had no long-term complications or issues due to his early start to life. Jack was in speech therapy for 2 years, but any issues have since resolved. He is an active kindergartner who loves to play with Legos, draw, and ice-skate. Jack has a fondness for music and has even started taking guitar lessons. When we tell people that Jack was a preemie, most are surprised because of how well he is doing. We've come a long way from the long days in the NICU and will forever be grateful to the medical team that helped Jack and us.

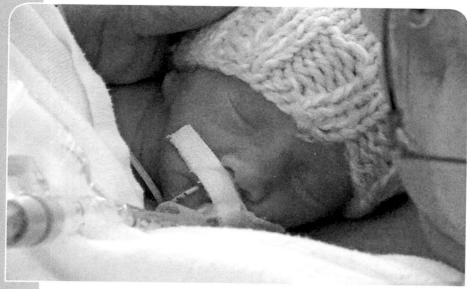

Jack was born at 29 weeks' gestation in 2009.

Henry

- Born in 2012, 2 years and 3 months after his brother Jack
- Weight: 3 pounds 7 ounces
- Gestational age: 31 weeks
- NICU stay: 47 days

Henry was born with issues common for a baby at his gestation, mainly breathing. He was on continuous positive airway pressure (CPAP) for a short time and was able to wean to a nasal cannula after a few days. Henry's course in the NICU was uneventful when compared to our other son, Jack, which we were grateful for. He went home without oxygen and no specialist follow-up. Today, Henry is a rambunctious 3½-year-old. He is definitely our "active" child who loves to run and play sports. He started soccer last fall and will continue this spring. His favorite sports are soccer, baseball, and ice-skating. He has no long-term complications or issues due to his early start. He is currently in speech therapy but has progressed quickly and will be stopping soon. As with Jack, we are amazed and forever grateful to the wonderful medical team and staff during Henry's stay in the NICU.

Kristina, mother of Jack and Henry

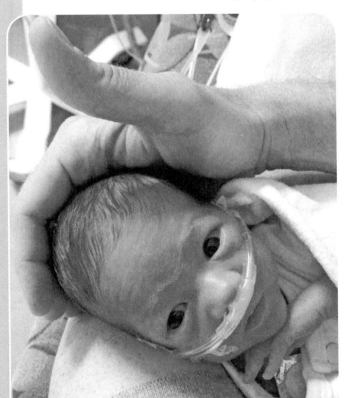

Henry was born at 31 weeks' gestation in 2012.

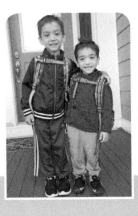

Jack, at age 6 years, and his brother, Henry, at age 3½ years.

CHAPTER 10

As Your Child Grows

"Looking back now, it was truly amazing to see him develop and grow before our eyes and get stronger each day. We were growing as parents too, even though we were thrown into the deep end of the pool and had to paddle to survive."

*Amanda, mother of **Maxwell***

The neonatal intensive care unit (NICU) experience doesn't end when you arrive home. Many parents describe their baby's first year of life as the longest roller-coaster ride of their lives. The first weeks at home are filled with mixed emotions, new challenges, and changes within your family. Now that you're home and settled into a routine, you'll begin looking to the future.

"Will My Baby Be Normal?"

Having a baby in the NICU can be a frightening experience, and your initial concerns may have focused on whether your baby would survive. Once your baby is medically stable, though, it's only natural to wonder, "Will my baby be normal?" Knowing what kind of follow-up to expect for your baby and how you can contribute to your baby's progress are rewarding aspects of parenting a NICU graduate.

You play an extremely important role in your baby's growth and development. Loving interactions shared with attentive parents can help babies who were born preterm, at risk, or with certain neonatal problems achieve optimum development. This chapter addresses how to monitor your baby's development and things you can do to help your baby reach his potential.

Risk Factors

Many parents worry about their baby's risk of ongoing health problems, possible physical challenges, and learning delays. Studies show that NICU graduates do have a higher risk of health issues and learning or developmental delays during infancy and early childhood compared with babies who do not need NICU care. Usually, the lower a newborn's birth weight and the more complicated the hospital stay, the greater the risk of future problems.

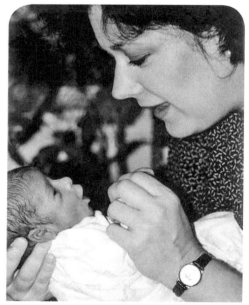

Take advantage of the moments when your baby is alert to talk to him, sing songs, and socialize.

Some of the factors that put babies at higher risk are a birth weight less than 1,500 g (3 lb 5 oz), also called very low birth weight; brain injury (bleeding in the brain or damage to the developing nervous system); poor head growth; chronic lung disease (bronchopulmonary dysplasia); serious vision loss; certain genetic syndromes; and abnormal muscle tone (remarkably weak or stiff muscles).

Parenting and the Learning Environment

Of course, a baby's medical problems are not the only factors determining his developmental outcome. Your baby's environment plays a big part in his health and learning. Supportive parenting and an environment rich in learning opportunities are important for every baby's growth and development.

The amount of attention, stimulation, and opportunities to learn new skills that a baby receives at home plays a part in the baby's developmental outcome.

This does not mean you have to buy expensive toys that claim to make babies smarter. Your baby needs to be loved and nurtured. Babies can learn a lot from the people around them and from an environment that's naturally rich with learning opportunities for a curious mind. Simple activities that you share with your baby, like talking, singing, reading a book, and imitating each other's facial expressions, provide the stimulation needed to help your baby reach his developmental potential.

Developmental Milestones and Your Baby

Developmental milestones are the skills or achievements that your baby develops in steps as he grows. For example, typical milestones that you will watch for include social skills, like making eye contact and smiling; large muscle (motor) skills, like bringing his hands to his mouth; and small muscle skills, like grasping objects. Developmental milestones follow patterns that you can monitor. Typically, babies develop large muscle skills from the head down. For example, babies usually develop head control before they learn to roll over or sit.

Watching for Progress

It is a good idea to keep your own record of your baby's progress. When trying to spot a delay in developing milestones, it is helpful to know the signs of typical development. Many baby books describe infant development and have places to keep track of developmental milestones. The American Academy of Pediatrics official Web site for parents, **www.HealthyChildren.org**, has an online tool that includes an interactive checklist of milestones that teaches parents more about physical development in babies and young children. It can serve as a guide if you have a feeling that something is wrong, and you can print a checklist of items to start a conversation with your pediatrician. There are also links to other reliable sites, such as the Centers for Disease Control and Prevention (**www.cdc.gov/milestones**) and Pathways.org (**www.pathways.org**),that provide checklists to help you track your baby's progress and suggest games and activities to stimulate development. Whether you use a book or an online checklist, bring your record to all of your follow-up appointments so information can be shared with your pediatrician or developmental specialist.

When you watch your baby's development, remember to adjust your baby's age for his preterm birth to get a better sense of where he should be in his development. For example, if your baby is 6 months old (24 weeks) but he was born 10 weeks early, his corrected age is 14 weeks (24 weeks minus 10 weeks = 14 weeks). This means you should be looking at the milestones listed under the 3- to 4-month (12–16 week) section. Use this corrected age when you look at developmental milestones for the first 2 years of your child's life. (See Chapter 9 for more information about corrected age.)

As you watch your baby's development, remember that babies follow similar patterns but do not always learn the same things at the same times. Babies develop skills at their own pace and may reach milestones in different ways. Even healthy term babies achieve developmental milestones over a range of ages. Some babies are walking by 9 months; others, not until 15 months. This will be especially true for preterm babies. Some babies are more assertive, more active, and quicker to learn, and, therefore, may develop at a faster pace than babies who are content to observe and quietly socialize.

Another important factor in developmental progress is the presence of chronic illness. Even if brain development is normal, babies with severe lung disease, heart disease, or intestinal problems may have delays because they cannot physically handle some activities. This is especially apparent in the baby's large muscle development.

Your baby may not meet each of the developmental milestones at the time described on the checklist. The most important thing is making sure your baby continues to make progress with his developmental milestones.

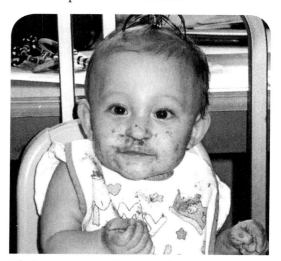 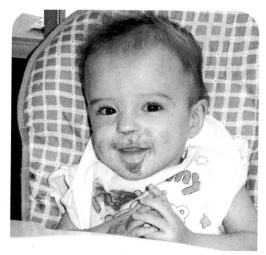

"I feel sad at moments like these, when my smooshy little babies seem too grown up. I feel sad because I didn't take enough time to enjoy them. Their babyhood was so full of overwhelming stress, anxiety, sadness, and worry that it was hard to keep my head above water. Looking back, I wish I had been able to spend less time worrying over every silly milestone and had just enjoyed the little snickerdoodles that they were."

*Billie, mother of **Holland** and **Eden***

Optimizing Your Baby's Development

Understanding Your Baby

Every baby is different and might achieve developmental milestones in different ways. Take time to think about your baby and answer the questions listed below in the box titled "Understanding Your Baby's Development." Your answers will help you understand your baby and how he is growing.

Understanding Your Baby's Development

- How does my baby let me know what he is thinking and feeling?

- How does my baby let me know when he's had enough and needs a nap?

- Is he naturally louder and more active, or is he naturally quieter and less active?

- How does my baby like to explore the world with his body? Does he prefer to use his fingers and hands (small muscles) or arms and legs (big muscles)?

- What kind of objects and activities interest him?

- How does my baby respond to new situations? Does he prefer to look around before he feels safe, or does he jump right in? Does he need frequent breaks from lots of sights and sounds, or does he stay calm?

- What are my baby's strengths?

- In what ways does he need more support?

Adapted from American Academy of Pediatrics. *Supporting You and Your Preemie: Milestone Guidelines for Premature Babies.* Elk Grove Village, IL; American Academy of Pediatrics; 2008.

Things You Can Do

You are your baby's most important teacher. As your baby grows, you will have many opportunities to teach different skills. You will learn to couple realistic expectations of your baby's abilities with support and inspiration for your baby to stretch those abilities to his greatest potential. Suggestions for how to foster your baby's development are included in the box on the next page, titled "Ways to Optimize Your Baby's Development." If many of these suggestions seem like simple common sense, you are already on the right track to optimizing your baby's development!

Ways to Optimize Your Baby's Development

- Talk, smile, make happy sounds, laugh, and socialize with your baby.
- Sing songs to your baby.
- Read books to your baby.
- Respond to your baby's smile or babbling with your own smile, touch, or voice.
- Change your baby's position during play, including sitting and lying on his back or stomach.
- Offer toys and objects that your baby has to reach for.
- Bring your baby's hands together to the center of his body and allow your baby to bring his hands to his mouth.
- When your baby can hold objects, encourage him to makes sounds by banging objects together.
- When your baby is approaching 6 months' corrected age, place him on his back and place toys out of his reach on one side to encourage rolling onto his stomach.
- When your baby is approaching 9 months' corrected age, play social games (patty-cake) and name objects in his sight to encourage vocabulary development.
- Praise and encourage your baby's efforts.

Developmental Follow-up

At the time of discharge from the NICU, you and your baby may be referred to a developmental follow-up clinic at the same hospital or a different one in the region. You may also be given a

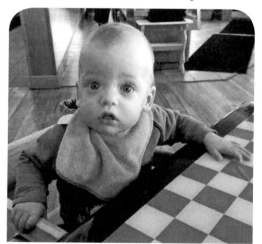

referral to your community early intervention program. Your pediatrician will be monitoring your baby's development and making any necessary referrals.

In the developmental follow-up clinic, you may see several specialists with knowledge about different aspects of growth and development. The specialists will look at how your baby moves, plays, and interacts with them. Similar to the list you use at home, the specialists use a variety of screening tests to score your baby's activity.

When **Auggie** goes to a restaurant to eat a meal with his parents, he has the opportunity to learn about his environment and to expand his vocabulary and social skills.

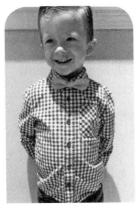

"When **Kellan** was 2 years old, our doctor told us that, on average, 2-year-olds should have a vocabulary of around 50 words. Kellan had about 10 words. We were shocked. Our pediatrician assured us that even though Kellan had not been accepted into the early intervention program a year ago, we should call and have him evaluated again. The speech therapist came to our house, and after the evaluation, we were excited to hear her say, 'I can't wait to work with Kellan.' She came to our house once a month for a year and Kellan went from 10 words to speaking in full sentences in no time. This picture was taken shortly after Kellan turned 3 and graduated from his therapy and headed off to preschool."

*Marnie, mother of **Kellan***

Individuals With Disabilities Education Act and Early Intervention

Because the foundation for learning begins in early infancy, every baby identified as at risk for developmental delay should receive intervention as early as possible. The Individuals With Disabilities Education Act is a law that ensures children with disabilities receive important services, including support and assistance for the family. The Early Intervention (EI) program is a federal grant run by individual states that works with children up to age 3 years who are at risk for developmental delays.

Your baby may be eligible for services if he experiences any difficulties with physical, mental, language, social, hearing, visual, behavioral, or emotional skills. Anyone can refer a child to the local EI program. You may have received a referral before your baby was discharged from the hospital, or your pediatrician may make a referral if any developmental concerns arise during office visits. You can even refer your baby to your local EI program by going to **www.cdc.gov/findEI** or calling 800/CDC-INFO (800/232-4636) and asking how to contact your state's EI program.

Once a referral is made, the EI program team of specialists will gather information about your baby and family to determine your needs. If the team determines your baby needs services, an Individualized Family Service Program (IFSP) will be developed. The IFSP explains the services that are recommended for your baby and how the EI program will help. Depending on your baby's needs, services such as occupational therapy, physical therapy, speech therapy, social work, or nursing care may be provided in your home or at a center. Your IFSP should be reviewed by you and your service coordinator at least every 6 months and modified as your child's needs change. You may request a review earlier if you feel your child needs more services or has outgrown his need for therapy. If your child still needs therapy when he turns 3 years old, he will transition from EI and an IFSP to an Individualized Education Program (IEP) and preschool services through your local school system.

Payment for EI services varies from state to state, but all states must provide at least some services free of charge. You can get information about your state EI program from your pediatrician, your state's department of health, your local health district, or the Early Childhood Technical Assistance Center Web site (**http://ectacenter.org**).

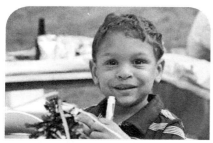

"At age 3, **Nathan** is developmentally on schedule in most areas and a joy in our life."

*Cheryl, mother of **Nathan***

Professionals can teach you developmentally appropriate activities to play with your baby. They may teach you special exercises to strengthen your baby's muscles or positioning techniques if your baby has any physical disabilities. Enjoy working with your baby, and take pride in knowing you are making a difference in his development.

Problems That May Worry You

As babies gets older, some may face ongoing developmental or physical challenges. Although many NICU graduates have no long-term health or developmental problems, it is important to know the types of problems that some NICU graduates have so you can watch for them and intervene early. Work with your child's pediatrician, therapists, and teachers to identify any areas of concern and find the right resources for help. You are not alone.

Learning Problems

Some NICU graduates experience learning problems, including problems with drawing and writing, language development, following directions, and reading comprehension. Children who experience these problems in school may require special education classes to assist their learning. Almost half of very low birth weight babies receive some form of special education in school. The percentage of babies diagnosed with intellectual disability increases as gestational age and birth weight decreases. At school age, very preterm babies have 2- to 5-times higher risk of having an intellectual disability compared with a healthy full-term baby, but the type of disability ranges widely from very mild to severe. Attempting to predict whether a baby will have an intellectual disability at school age is difficult when the baby is very young. A variety of developmental testing tools are available to evaluate older infants and toddlers.

Cerebral Palsy

Cerebral palsy (CP) is a diagnosis that many parents of preterm babies fear. It is an abnormality of muscle movement or tone caused by a malformation or damage to the nerve cells in the brain. Babies with CP have muscles that are too stiff or too limp and have poor coordination. The frequency of CP is higher in the smallest and most preterm babies and occurs in approximately 1 in 10 babies born weighing less than 1,500 g (3 lb 5 oz).

Cerebral palsy does not mean there is a problem with intelligence, although some children with CP will also have learning disabilities. The diagnosis of CP is generally not made until the preterm infant is 12 to 18 months' corrected age unless the infant's problems are severe. In some infants, muscle tone is increased (called *spasticity* or *hypertonia*); in others, muscles are abnormally limp (*hypotonia*). *Spastic diplegia,* or stiff muscle tone of the legs and arms, with more involvement of legs and feet, is the most common form of CP among preterm infants. Many preterm infants with this type of CP have normal to near-normal intelligence. *Spastic quadriplegia* is when all 4 extremities, along with the head and trunk, are fairly equally affected. This is the most severe form of CP and can often be diagnosed before the first year of life. Spastic quadriplegia is frequently associated with intellectual disability. As you can see, the characteristics of CP can range from mild muscle tone abnormalities with normal or above-average intelligence to severe physical and intellectual disability.

Signs of CP can vary because of the different types and degree of disability. Some of the early clues your baby may have CP focus on delays in achieving motor milestones. Some of the early warning signs are included in the box below, titled "Warning Signs of Cerebral Palsy." When looking at your baby for these signs, be sure to use his age corrected for prematurity.

Warning Signs of Cerebral Palsy

Younger than 6 months
- When cradled in your arms, he always acts as if he is pushing away from you, overextending his back and neck.
- When you pick him up, his legs get stiff and they cross each other or "scissor."

6 to 10 months old
- He reaches out with only one hand while keeping the other hand fisted.

Older than 10 months
- He is lopsided when crawling, pushing off with only one hand and leg while dragging the opposite hand and leg.
- He scoots around on his buttocks but does not crawl on all fours.

Adapted from American Academy of Pediatrics. *Caring for Your Baby and Young Child: Birth to Age 5.* Shelov SP, Altmann TR, 5th ed. New York, NY: Bantam Books; 2009.

Children diagnosed with CP need close developmental follow-up and referrals to an EI program. In addition to a developmental pediatrician, children with CP may be referred to pediatric neurology (brain), orthopedic (bone and joint), and physical medicine/rehabilitation specialists to plan their treatment.

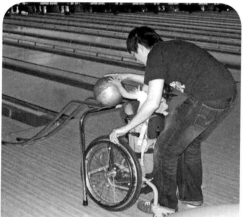

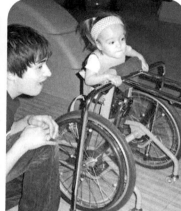

"We took the kids bowling today and had a lot of fun. I had the idea that Eden could bowl in her stander, and John noticed some kids bowling with one of these ramps. It worked out GREAT! **Eden** bowled an 87 and **Holland** a 105. They both bowled over my average."

Billie, mother of ***Holland*** *and* ***Eden***

> I've been thinking, pondering, wondering...how do I teach Eden that she is just like everyone else? That her disability does not define her? That she can do whatever she wants, based on her strengths? That everyone has strengths and weaknesses?
>
> How do I teach others that she is a 'normal' kid? That she should be treated the same as everyone else? That she loves all the same things that the other kids like? That she wants to play too?
>
> Then it hit me...she is NOT like everyone else.
>
> If I fail to recognize and accept her differences...if I fail to recognize and embrace her many strengths, I am failing her. She is different. Just like everyone else.
>
> Billie, mother of **Holland** and **Eden**

Vision and Hearing Problems

Graduates from the NICU, especially the tiniest and most preterm babies, are at risk for future vision and hearing problems.

Babies with severe retinopathy of prematurity (ROP) have the highest risk of serious vision problems. Even though most babies with ROP get better over time and never need treatment, a small number of preterm babies lose their vision from ROP. Continued follow-up with your eye doctor until the ROP is fully resolved is extremely important to prevent serious visual loss or blindness.

Babies born very preterm also have an increased risk of nearsightedness and crossed or lazy eyes in childhood. The risk is highest in babies who previously had severe ROP or significant bleeding in their brain. Because vision is so important for achieving developmental milestones, babies with visual problems need evaluation by a pediatric eye doctor (ophthalmologist), developmental follow-up, and EI.

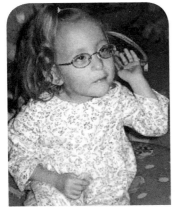

"Holland is awfully cute in her new pink glasses. She looks so grown-up and studious. We could tell when she first put them on that she knew something was different."

Billie, mother of **Holland** *and* **Eden**

Graduates from the NICU also have a higher risk of hearing loss. Even though studies show hearing loss is much more common in preterm babies compared with full-term babies, the chance is quite small. Between 1 and 4 of every 100 very preterm babies will have serious hearing loss requiring a hearing aid. Hearing problems can also occur in babies who had persistent pulmonary hypertension of the newborn, hypoxic-ischemic encephalopathy, severe jaundice (hyperbilirubinemia), or infections or who received medications that can affect the ear (certain antibiotics and diuretics). All NICU graduates have their hearing screened before hospital discharge, but hearing loss may not be discovered until later. If you have any concerns that your baby is not hearing normally, talk with your pediatrician.

Behavior Problems

Not all preterm or chronically ill babies have behavior problems in childhood, but some do. Babies who were born preterm or have been chronically ill may be less able to handle stimulation and show unpredictable feeding, crying, and sleeping patterns. Behavior problems seen in early childhood include frequent temper tantrums, overaggressiveness in play, hyperactivity, and exaggerated separation anxiety. Children may be extra-sensitive to loud sounds or certain textures that are touched or eaten. They may require parents to learn their special behavioral cues to prevent overstimulation.

As these children reach school age, their behaviors may worsen or improve with maturity. Some children have discipline problems because of a short attention span, hyperactivity, and disorganized behavior. Others may show more introverted behavior, with extreme shyness and anxiety.

If your child develops behavioral problems, close follow-up and teamwork with your pediatrician and schoolteachers is important to help your child reach his full potential.

Allowing Your NICU Graduate to Grow Up

Graduates of the NICU may come home with nursing support, equipment, supplies, medications, and a long list of caregiving requirements. You may have been given a list of dos and don'ts for your baby's care and warned of the potential for rehospitalization. It's no wonder that at first, you tend to overprotect your baby. In some cases, though, this sheltering continues well past the point of necessity and beyond what is healthy for you and your child.

Vulnerable Child Syndrome

When parents continue to view their child as sickly despite healthy findings on physical examinations, these parents may be experiencing something called *vulnerable child syndrome*. When the child reaches school age, these parents do not allow participation in sports or special events. The parents don't encourage high academic standards, and so their healthy child performs below his potential.

Overprotection stunts children's efforts to develop skills appropriate for their age. They may continue to experience separation anxiety and have temper tantrums whenever they do not get their way. They may have difficulty playing with or participating in games with other children. They may bite or hit other children during outbursts of anger.

Professional intervention is often necessary to help parents recognize and accept that the illness event, which took place years earlier, is now over. Only then can these parents begin to view their child as a healthy individual and encourage his social development.

A Difficult Balance

Because your baby spent time in the NICU, he is at risk for being overprotected. Close watchfulness may be necessary and appropriate early in life because of continued medical problems. Listen to your pediatrician and other child care specialists when they tell you your baby is medically stable and developmentally ready for new challenges. They can educate you about normal baby behavior and basic parenting.

Caring for and protecting your baby without providing too much care and protection is, indeed, a tricky balancing act. You've worked hard to get to this point, and it's only natural to want to safeguard your special baby. But part of being a parent is growing with your child and realizing when it's time to loosen your grip in some areas and to expect your child's cooperation in others.

As your child explores the world and begins to feel accomplished as an individual, he will grow healthier. You'll find your own way as you give your child's potential abilities a chance to unfold. Through trial and error, you'll learn how much to expect from your child and when the time is right to stretch your expectations a bit further. Every child's needs are different, but most benefit from parents who expect accomplishments that reflect their child's fullest abilities.

Working With Your Pediatrician

Remember that you are not alone. Your pediatrician is your partner and is dedicated to helping you meet your child's health and developmental needs. If you have concerns about your child,

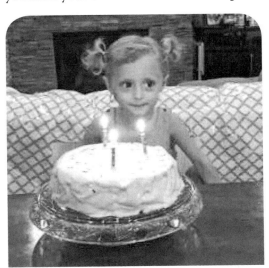

start by talking with your pediatrician. You may be asked to complete some additional screening questionnaires. Your observations are an important part of your pediatrician's evaluation. If a specific diagnosis is found, your pediatrician can help you to connect with resources or special support groups in your community.

"I rarely refer to her as a preemie. She was born a preemie, but she is all toddler now."

*Lisa, mother of **Frankie***

Believing in Yourself

Many parents of NICU graduates are a bit frightened to look far ahead. In fact, fear of the unknown contributes to chronic stress in many families. The potential for rehospitalization, future health problems, and overprotection of your child is very real.

The NICU experience does not make for an easy transition to parenthood. As your baby grows, you'll continue to discover important parenting resources within yourself—for managing stress, advocating for your baby's needs, and seeking support and lending it to those around you. For you, parenthood has brought with it unique changes that are different from those felt by parents whose baby was born healthy. It's given you opportunities for strengthening relationships, uncovering hidden strengths, and reordering priorities.

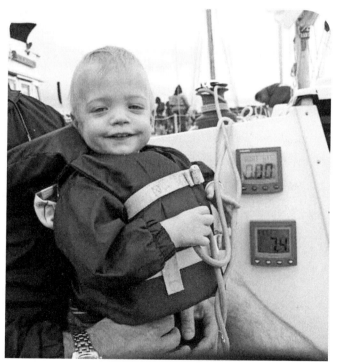

"Auggie had his first boating adventure at about 18 months. He thoroughly enjoyed it."

*Robyn, mother of **Auggie***

Talking to Your Pediatrician About Your Baby's Development

Helpful tips

- When making the appointment, tell the office staff that you have concerns about your baby's development and want to discuss them with the doctor.

- Bring a list of your questions, concerns, and any examples you can think of.

- Fill out one of the milestone checklists from the American Academy of Pediatrics official Web site for parents, **www.HealthyChildren.org**; Pathways.org (**www.pathways.org**), or Centers for Disease Control and Prevention (**www.cdc.gov/milestones**).

- Ask another adult who knows your child to fill out the milestone checklist too.

- If you can, take another adult with you to play with your child so you can focus on what your doctor says.

Ask all of your questions during the visit.

- Tell your doctor that you have concerns right at the start of the visit and share the checklist and questions that you wrote down.

- If your doctor is in a hurry on that day, ask if you can schedule another visit.

- Ask your doctor about the results of the most recent developmental screening.

- Takes notes to help you remember what your doctor says.

Make sure you understand the next steps.

- Before you leave, make sure your questions have been answered.

- If you don't understand something, ask your doctor to explain it again or in a different way.

- Make sure you know the next steps and have the information you need. For example, do you need to make an appointment with a specialist? Do you have the phone number? Do you need a written referral?

- Review your notes when you get home and call the doctor's office if you have more questions.

Adapted from Centers for Disease Control and Prevention. Learn the Signs. Act Early. **http://www.cdc.gov/actearly**. Accessed June 28, 2016.

You may face many challenges ahead. But you can feel good about your abilities as a parent as long as you continue to ask questions and actively participate on the health care team as your baby's advocate.

Your baby's growth and development will reflect not only his medical legacy, but the way you bring him up, as well. A parent's most difficult task is knowing when to offer a helping hand—and when to provide a gentle push forward. Your job is to inspire achievement and independence, while realizing that some of life's most valuable lessons come from disappointment. Your success as a parent depends on your ability to trust yourself to have a positive effect on your child's life.

Your child's success will depend largely on your outlook on life and what you teach him about achieving his personal best. The NICU experience creates unique challenges for parents and babies. Take a moment to congratulate yourself for a job well done.

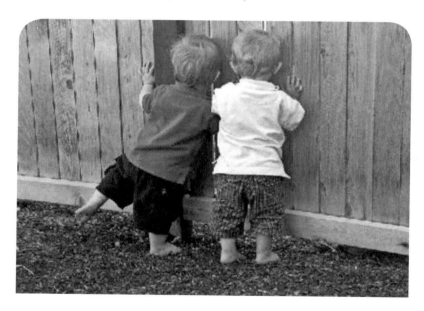

The next chapter discusses the loss of a baby. The neonatal intensive care unit is a place of remarkable healing and recovery, and most babies do not die there. But, sometimes, despite everything, a baby will not live. We are so sorry if this has happened to you and your family. We are honored and grateful to Adrienne for sharing her memories in the following chapter. Even though your experience will be yours alone, we hope that her insight and advice will support you as you learn what to expect as your own story unfolds.

"A nurse sat in the room with us
and it was very peaceful and quiet.
Clara breathed for a while
and then her breaths
became inconsistent.
Slowly she went away.
The very last thing
I remember about her
was a tiny tear that slid
down her face and then
she was gone."

*Adrienne, mother of **Clara***

CHAPTER 11

The Loss of Your Baby

"Remembering the day Clara was born
is something I don't do very much
anymore. We had an unplanned home
birth after a very fast labor, and for
some reason, she never breathed.
She made it to the NICU, but the next
day the doctors explained that she was
not going to live. When I think of Clara,
I do it with great care and
affection. I've come to accept
her short life and have stopped
questioning why."

Adrienne, mother of **Clara**

There are few experiences in life as difficult as the heartbreaking death of a baby. As parents, you must face the loss of your baby and your dreams. You might also have to manage the practical details of the situation while continuing to support others who rely on you. This experience will change who you are and how you live. As this experience unfolds, please remember that *you* are your baby's parent. Although the opportunities to parent your baby may have been limited or very different from what you hoped, you will participate in the important decisions that affect you and your baby. Everything you do will help create the memory you will have for the rest of your life.

Difficult Choices for a Seriously Ill Baby

The birth of an extremely preterm baby or a baby with a significant birth defect frequently raises many questions and requires parents to make difficult decisions. If the problem is known before your baby's birth, your doctors will have the chance to meet with you and have a detailed discussion about the potential health problems your baby is expected to have and what treatment options are available. Sometimes, a preterm birth happens quickly. Sometimes, a serious birth defect isn't discovered until after birth or a baby develops a life-threatening complication, and you will have an unexpected discussion with your baby's doctors. This can be very frightening. In either case, parents may have to make difficult choices about their baby's care.

Often, the outcome (*prognosis*) is not as certain, and the NICU team will work with you to make the best decisions for your baby's care. A baby may have problems that would require prolonged and uncomfortable treatment but still have only a small chance of survival. If the baby does survive, she may have serious disabilities that would require lifelong care and limit her ability to enjoy everyday activities. In this case, you will work with the health care team to make very difficult decisions. The doctors, nurses, and other health care team members will provide you with as much information as possible about your baby's condition and her prognosis. The NICU team will explain your baby's problems, with their best estimate of what she would require to survive, risks of the treatment, and different possible outcomes. Some families put the highest value on any chance of their baby's survival, even if it means their baby could endure a long hospitalization, multiple procedures, and possibly survive with serious disabilities. Other families choose to spend a short amount of time

> ❝ Our voice was honored all the way through. After Clara was admitted to the NICU, I needed surgery, so I couldn't be with Clara the night she was born, but my husband and his sister were with her. The NICU allowed them to do what they needed to move through this experience. They allowed them to take pictures, stay with her, talk to her, have her baptized....They supported our process without inserting their own agenda. The NICU staff remained silently supportive. ❞
>
> Adrienne, mother of **Clara**

with their baby, without medical devices, and limit the possibility of pain and suffering. Working together, your NICU team will be there for you to discuss your thoughts, your questions, and your beliefs and decide what type of treatment is best for your baby.

Together, you may decide to continue intensive life-sustaining treatment, to continue certain treatments but not others, or to stop life-sustaining treatment and focus on providing comfort and pain relief to your baby. If you decide to put limits on which treatments you want, the doctor may ask you to help write a care plan so all of your baby's caregivers know your wishes and goals and what treatments are acceptable. A *do not resuscitate* or *DNR order* may be part of that plan. A DNR order indicates you do not want emergency measures, like chest compressions (CPR) or emergency medications (such as epinephrine), used if your baby's heart stops beating or she stops breathing.

The decision to stop life-sustaining treatment and allow a baby to die comfortably is not made by a single person or by the parents alone. Like you, the NICU team wants what is best for your baby, and your input is essential. It is important that you understand the available treatment options and the possible risks and benefits of each option and carefully consider what you believe is best for your baby. In most cases, there is no single right answer. Even though the NICU team may have faced a similar situation before, each baby and family are unique. Two families faced with the same situation may make completely different choices. What is most important is that you feel the decisions were right for your baby.

Considering the Decision to Stop Life-sustaining Therapy

When the NICU team asks to talk with you about making treatment decisions that include the possibility of stopping life-sustaining treatment, you may not be ready. You may even be shocked or angry that they asked. When facing this situation, ask as many questions as you need to, and then ask again to make sure you understand the answers. Some questions do not have answers, but the team will try to explain everything they can. You will find some suggestions to help you with this conversation on the next page.

Parents often feel a sense of relief after they reach agreement about such a difficult decision. At times, you will likely second-guess your decision and have some doubts, but these are normal feelings that will take time, and sometimes professional help, to resolve. This will certainly be one of the hardest experiences you will ever go through, but you will not regret taking part in the decision-making process. If you and the NICU team determine that intensive medical treatment is prolonging suffering without any benefit, care for your baby will shift to providing as much support and comfort as possible. Allowing your baby to have a peaceful and comfortable death is a choice that you make as loving parents who only want the best for your baby.

When Parents Have to Make Difficult Decisions

- Avoid getting critical information about your baby over the phone.

- Write down your questions as you think of them so you don't forget to ask later.

- Let the NICU team know who you would like to be with you during difficult conversations. Is there someone in your family or a support person you want to be with you? Are there topics that you don't want discussed in front of family members?

- If your baby's condition has a name, ask your doctor to write it down for you. You can ask what caused the problem. Sometimes, it is not any one specific condition that has led to your baby's critical situation but a series of complications resulting from the original problem.

- Ask your doctor to explain the condition. What are the treatment choices? Can the outcome of each choice be predicted?

- If necessary, remind the NICU team to use words that you understand and to talk at a pace that allows you to consider the information and ask questions.

- Tell your NICU team if there are cultural or religious factors that influence your decision-making process or practices that are important to you in this situation.

- Take your time. Let your doctor know when you are overwhelmed with information and need a break. This also gives you time to think of questions and write them down.

- Repeat the information in your own words to make sure you understand what you have been told.

- If English is not your preferred language, ask for a medical translator. Do not use a family member, a friend, or a child to translate.

- In some cases, your doctor may be able to connect you to a family who has faced a similar decision and can provide some additional perspective for your decision-making.

Organ Donation

Organ donation may be a way of having something good come out of this terrible experience. Although it will not bring your baby back to you, it may allow someone else's baby to live. Neonatal organ donation is a very personal and emotional decision.

If your baby is dying and you would like to donate her organs, talk to your baby's doctor. Babies who die in the NICU may not be eligible to become organ donors because of their size or the time between stopping life support and the baby's death. Your doctor will contact the agency responsible for organ donation in your area and find out if your baby meets the criteria. If she does, a counselor from the organ donation agency will talk with you about the possibility.

Preparing to Say Farewell

You may feel very alone during this time, but you will probably be surrounded by loved ones who are also experiencing this loss with you. Your own parents, grandparents, older children, and close friends and other relatives may grieve with you.

Reuniting Mother and Baby

If your baby was transported to another hospital, both parents may not be with her when difficult decisions are made or when she is near death. Ask your NICU team what can be done to get mother and baby together. If you are the mother and you are medically stable, an early hospital discharge may be arranged. If your insurance allows, a mother may also be medically transferred to the hospital where her baby is receiving care.

Naming Your Baby

If you have not yet done so, consider giving your baby a name. Naming your baby will help you and others recognize that your baby has a place in the story of your life. Naming your baby also establishes a memory that you will be able to reflect on later. Referring to a baby by name, even after death, gives dignity to that life.

Family Participation

The NICU staff will encourage family members, including older siblings, to be together as a family when a baby dies. Spending time with your baby gives family members the opportunity to know her and have their own memories. This is also the opportunity to incorporate your family traditions or spiritual customs into your baby's life. With your permission, religious clergy are always welcome in the NICU. The hospital's chaplaincy service can accommodate many different traditions and may be able to help if you prefer clergy of a specific denomination.

Events may occur quickly. Birth, death, and funeral may occupy only a few days. Experiencing this tragedy as a family will help everyone get through it. In addition, when the family talks about the baby in the future, all family members who participated will be able to share their memories and support.

Bringing Your Baby Home to Die

Not all babies with incurable conditions require a lot of technological support. You may consider taking your baby home to die. If you are considering this, talk with your NICU team about what you would like to do and learn about the rules and regulations that affect your options. If it is possible to take your baby home to die and you decide to do so, the NICU team will help you develop a home care plan, teach you what to expect as your baby's condition changes, and provide a contact person who will be available at all times to answer questions and give support.

Near the Time of Death

When your baby is dying, the main priority is the baby's comfort and companionship. If you are in the NICU, the staff will make arrangements for you to hold your baby, preferably in a private, quiet area. Many of the tubes, wires, and medical equipment may have been removed so you can hold your baby closely without interference. This may be the first time you are able to hold and care for your baby without wires and tubes getting in the way.

The NICU team will tell you and your partner what you can expect to see, hear, and feel as you hold your baby. You may ask your nurse to stay with you or just to be available if you call. This is important parenting time, so do not feel pressured or hurried. Someone from the NICU team will listen to your baby's heartbeat every so often with a stethoscope to determine the time of death. Sometimes, babies will die very quickly after life support equipment is removed, but other times, babies will have a slow heartbeat and take occasional breaths for a long time. While comforting your baby, let your nurse know if you need to take a break.

> The role the nurses, doctors, and social workers played at the hospital was significant. Our ability to move through this experience in the most positive way was made possible by their nurturing and guidance. They took the best care of Clara and all of us. They guided our decisions with their knowledge and experience and captured the important memories for us to hold onto. My entire family is forever thankful and we still remember everyone at the hospital with the fondest of memories.
>
> Adrienne, mother of **Clara**

Preparing Memories

The NICU staff will help your family prepare memories of your baby. Many parents want to take photographs and hold their baby for a family portrait. Some NICUs have an arrangement with a hospital-based or professional photographer specially trained to take these photos. Tell your nurse if you have special clothes or a blanket that you want your baby wrapped in for the photos. Some families think they don't want photos or aren't ready to take them home right away. You can still ask the staff to take photographs and save them at the hospital until you are ready to receive them some time after your baby's death.

> " We still have the memory book with her hair and prints and measurements. It brings such joy to my heart knowing that the nurses took the time to record her short life and treat her so well. "
>
> Adrienne, mother of **Clara**

Many NICUs will help you prepare a memory box including such things as the blankets and clothing you brought in, footprints, the hospital ID bracelet, a tape measure, the baby's crib card, and even a lock of hair. You may find all of this comforting, but if you do not, consider keeping these items in case you decide you want them later on.

After Death

After your baby has died, you still have all the time you need to say good-bye. When you are ready, your baby's nurse will undress your baby and prepare her to be carried to the hospital morgue. It is common for nurses to bathe the baby before leaving the NICU, and you are welcome to help or give the bath yourself. Doing something like this for your baby may help you say good-bye, but don't feel you must if it makes you uncomfortable. After the bath, you may want to rock and hold your baby again. After you have said good-bye, your baby will receive special identification tags and be carried to the morgue.

> ❝ Depending on your situation, this might be the only time you will ever spend with your baby. Take the time to hold, look at, and talk to your baby. Take pictures. You don't want to rush through this because when you look back, these memories will be all you have. I can't stress this enough, as it is my big and only regret. I was too quick to end the moment because it was so painful. When I look back and when we celebrate Clara's birthdays, the only wish I have is that I would have sat with her longer, talked to her, and been with her longer. In fact, when asked if there was one wish I could have come true, that wish is to go back and sit in that room with her one more time. ❞
>
> Adrienne, mother of **Clara**

Taking the Next Steps

After your baby has died, you and your partner will be asked to consider some additional choices. If you are having trouble, call on those who have helped and supported you up until now—your nurses, doctors, family, friends, social workers, and clergy.

Considering an Autopsy

After your baby dies, a member of the NICU team will ask you to consider an autopsy. An autopsy, or postmortem examination, can provide valuable information that helps you understand why your baby died and identify any additional problems that weren't known before death. Sometimes, the results will provide information that might be useful when thinking about future pregnancies for you or your relatives.

If your baby died in a small hospital, your doctor may ask to have the autopsy performed at a neighboring medical center or children's hospital. The early results may be known in a few days, but the detailed results can take 6 weeks or more. Usually, the doctor who cared for your baby will meet with you, explain the results, and, if you wish, give you a copy of the report.

Funeral Arrangements and Transport

A funeral will let you, your family, and your close friends say good-bye to your baby in a public way as a celebration of your baby's short life. It also allows public recognition that this was a person who lived and had a profound influence on the lives she touched.

After your baby's death, you will be asked to identify a funeral home whose staff will help to make all of the other arrangements. Your NICU social worker, family support representative, or grief counselor may be able to provide a list of area funeral homes and other available resources. If you are not sure what kind of ceremony is right for you and your baby, talk with the professionals at the funeral home. If your baby dies far from where you live, the funeral home can help you arrange transport, if needed.

Talking With Friends

As painful as it may be, you'll need to tell your close friends what happened. If your baby's life was very short, friends may not even know that your baby was born. This may be your first chance to speak with them about your baby. Calling close friends helps mobilize support, validates your feelings of loss as they express their shock and grief, and helps you find a way to live with this loss. If you wish, ask family members or a few close friends to pass the news to other friends. This relieves you of endless phone calls.

Understanding Grief

It's important to recognize that no 2 people grieve the same way. Not everyone experiences all of the stages of the grief process, and people experiencing the same loss may not experience the stages at the same time or in the same way.

At this point in your life, it may seem that nothing will ever make you feel good again. No one can tell you exactly how to get through this experience, but you may find some of the following suggestions helpful. If you have previously experienced a loss or have survived crises before, try to recall what helped you most in that situation. Was it spending time with a friend? Attending a group session? Also, try to maintain your usual daily habits, even if you are unable to sleep. A sense of routine may help you feel more normal and less "lost."

Differences in How Partners Grieve

Men and women often grieve differently. Society expects men to be strong and unemotional in a crisis, while women are allowed to cry and "fall apart." Women may feel as though they have to take care of their mate, physically and emotionally. Men may become distant and quiet, unable to show emotions because it makes them too vulnerable. At times, fathers have been ignored during the grieving process because of the erroneous belief that they do not experience the same loss as mothers. Allowing fathers to grieve openly may help them resolve their grief.

Sometimes, one partner will return to work soon after the death of a baby. When they focus on their work, it may appear they are not grieving or have moved beyond their grief. Neither may be true. The difference may be that they are not alone all day long focusing on their grief. When they come home, they may need to set their own grief aside to provide support to a grieving partner or child.

Lack of communication between partners is one of the reasons for the high divorce rate among couples who have lost a baby. The loss of a baby may be the first major crisis a couple faces together. It can be frightening to see your partner lose control, and it may be difficult to deal with a crisis if both of you are lost, overwhelmed, and unable to support each other. The stress is great, and the potential for misunderstanding each other is high. It's helpful if couples talk over small misunderstandings before they become insurmountable problems.

Coping Strategies

During this time, you may find relief by expressing yourself artistically. This serves 2 purposes. First, it can help you sort through your emotions day by day. Second, when everything is over and for many years to come, your work will provide you with remembrances and memories of a bittersweet time. Some creative coping strategies include writing (for example, letters to your baby, poetry, a journal, blogging), scrapbooking, drawing, painting, creating pottery, or sculpting. It is entirely up to you whether you share these outlets or keep them private.

Some parents find comfort by joining a parent support group. Sometimes, talking to others who have experienced the same or similar event is very helpful. The NICU social worker can give you more information.

> " After Clara's funeral, they allowed me to come back and meet all of the nurses and doctors who tended to Clara in the NICU. That was a very healing day for me. I wanted to meet and talk to the people who spent more time with her than I did. They shared little tidbits and cared enough to tell me everything they could remember about Clara and how she may have touched their lives. I took the time to thank them and tell them I knew they did everything short of being God to keep her alive. I felt there wasn't a single thing that could have been done differently and that was so comforting. I would hate to be grieving while thinking there was something more that could have been done—that would have been torture. Their support went above and beyond any expectation I could have had. "
>
> Adrienne, mother of **Clara**

Loss of a Twin or Other Multiple

Multiple-gestation births can be a special event, but parents who lose one child from a set of twins or other multiple births face a unique situation. The loss of one child is not made up for by the survival of another. The child who is lost is always missed and always mourned, even if only privately.

Caring for the surviving twin may be a source of sadness and joy. Your emotions are on a roller-coaster ride as you celebrate the birth and life of a healthy baby and grieve for what has been lost. Because of the turmoil around the death of one baby, parents may feel like they are ignoring the needs of the other. They may feel guilty that they can only provide the basic needs of their other baby, such as feeding and diapering, but cannot attend to their emotional needs.

With time, a balance can be found. With time, many parents learn to be happy for the surviving baby and deal with that baby's problems while grieving for the baby who has died. Each parent reacts to the death of a multiple differently. The only way to get through the experience is to talk about it and respect each other's feelings.

Helping Others Cope With Grief

Coping with your own feelings may seem like all you can do right now, but as you move through your grief, you may find yourself supporting those around you.

Grandparents

Your baby's grandparents will grieve in their own ways for their own reasons. Like parents, they grieve the loss of the future. Grandparents develop their own fantasies about their grandchild—what the baby will look like, what they will do together, what they hope the baby will become. When a grandchild dies or is severely disabled, grandparents also mourn the loss of that future.

In addition, grandparents hurt for you, their own children. They never stop being parents, and your pain compounds their grief. But don't overlook the support your parents offer. They may be separated from the situation enough to help you make plans and decisions.

Your Baby's Siblings

Sibling grief reactions vary, depending on the age of the sibling. Although younger children may not fully comprehend what has occurred, even the youngest child will sense the emotional turmoil surrounding the loss of the baby. Unlike adults, children do not grieve continuously. Much to your surprise, your children may be able to continue their daily routine and play and eat as usual. Then, when you least expect it, one of them may remember something about the baby and become very sad.

Some predictable grief reactions occur in children. They may feel guilty because they believe they caused their sibling's death or disability by wishful thinking. They may misbehave and regress in their behavior (for example, go back to thumb-sucking or bed-wetting). They may experience frightening thoughts that others are going to die. They may also be frightened at the strong emotions they see from you for the first time.

When explaining death to children, use real words and express the problems honestly. Children may need reassurance that the same thing will not happen to them. Avoid talking about death as going to sleep; that may result in sleeping problems. Be honest: "The baby was born too soon and she was too small," "The baby's heart didn't work right and she couldn't make it," "The baby was born very sick and she died," and especially, "The baby's problems are nobody's fault."

Be as honest as possible with your children without going into too much detail. Answer questions concisely with as much explanation as you feel is appropriate. It's all right to admit that you don't have all the answers. Resources are available to assist you, but remember—you know your children best. Trust your instincts as you struggle with what to say.

Children are as unique as adults and may grieve in unique ways. An unconcerned attitude that continues without any change, however, may be a signal that your child is denying the situation or is unable to express his or her emotions. Your child may benefit from professional counseling in dealing with the feelings.

Friends

You may have friends who were—or are still—pregnant at this time. Seeing these friends can be especially challenging after your baby has died. Friends may respond to your loss in a number of ways. Some who are sad and scared for you may withdraw simply because they do not know what to do or say. Others may be more comfortable with your grief, stay close, and support you through this difficult time.

Many people have difficulty speaking to mourning parents and say nothing or the wrong thing. You will probably encounter many well-intentioned people with a knack for saying the wrong thing: "You're young; you can have others"; "This happened for the best"; and, "At least you still have one of the twins." You will probably also have dear, close friends who realize that saying "I'm sorry" or "We're thinking of you," or just their presence, is a great comfort to you.

Duration of Grief

Your life has now changed forever, but you will eventually find a new place of emotional peace where you feel comfortable and belong.

When to Get Help for Your Grief

Throughout the grief process, you may wonder if you are normal. You may wonder if you have been sad, angry, or feeling confused for too long. Most people are able to work through their grief with help from their partner, family members, friends, and coworkers. However, you may want to obtain help from a therapist, family counselor, social worker, or other professional if you feel you need it or if any of the following situations occur:

- You are afraid you may physically harm yourself or someone else; you have thoughts of suicide.
- You are participating in activities that may damage your health (for example, drugs, alcohol, overeating, not eating enough).
- The support of friends and family members is not enough.
- You experience more losses after the death of your baby.
- You think very poorly of yourself and feel out of control, depressed, or stressed out all the time.

People grieve at their own pace. The first year is usually one of experiencing all of the "firsts," living a full year of special dates (birthdays and holidays), and feeling the acute pain of your loss as these dates occur. Even though your baby's death may not affect how your family celebrates a particular event, you may feel your loss most at family gatherings.

The second year is usually spent looking toward the future, reorganizing your life without your baby in it. As time passes, your loss will feel less physically painful and you'll learn to laugh again. Expect to experience occasional "blue" days, when some date or event causes you to reexperience your grief. Your grief may come and go over time, and small remembrances may trigger strong feelings of grief again. If you feel you are too sad for too long, consider speaking with your own doctor or a mental health professional.

One of the most challenging considerations for parents who have lost a child is how to answer the innocent question, "How many children do you have?" Your answer to this question may change over time, and you may have different replies in different circumstances. This is completely acceptable, and you will learn what is most comfortable for you.

> We have another child, a boy, who was born 16 months after Clara. I have always felt her spirit in him, like a little dancing angel who twinkles through at the most unexpected times. I am at peace.
>
> Adrienne, mother of **Clara**

A Bittersweet Time

Few things in life are more difficult than making decisions for a critically ill or dying baby. Drawing on the love and support of family, friends, and the NICU health care team will help you make the choices that will ultimately be best for you and your child.

It may take time for your decisions to feel completely right. The choices facing you are complex and will awaken many new emotions. As time goes by, though, you'll be thankful you were empowered to make these choices for your baby and grateful you were able to control some aspects of this very overwhelming time in your life.

Appendix

To Convert Pounds and Ounces to Grams or Grams to Pounds and Ounces

Find the baby's weight in pounds down the left side of the table. Find the ounces across the top of the table. The intersection of the 2 measurements equals the equivalent weight in grams. For example, 3 pounds 8 ounces equals 1,588 g. To convert grams to pounds and ounces, find the baby's weight in grams. Look to the far left line for the pounds and to the top of the gram column for the ounces. For example, 1,134 g equals 2 pounds 8 ounces.

Conversion of Pounds and Ounces to Grams

Pounds \ Ounces	0	1	2	3	4	5	6	7	8	9	10	11	12	13	14	15
0	—	28	57	85	113	142	170	198	227	255	283	312	340	369	397	425
1	454	482	510	539	567	595	624	652	680	709	737	765	794	822	850	879
2	907	936	964	992	1,021	1,049	1,077	1,106	1,134	1,162	1,191	1,219	1,247	1,276	1,304	1,332
3	1,361	1,389	1,417	1,446	1,474	1,502	1,531	1,559	1,588	1,616	1,644	1,673	1,701	1,729	1,758	1,786
4	1,814	1,843	1,871	1,899	1,928	1,956	1,984	2,013	2,041	2,070	2,098	2,126	2,155	2,183	2,211	2,240
5	2,268	2,296	2,325	2,353	2,381	2,410	2,438	2,466	2,495	2,523	2,551	2,580	2,608	2,637	2,665	2,693
6	2,722	2,750	2,778	2,807	2,835	2,863	2,892	2,920	2,948	2,977	3,005	3,033	3,062	3,090	3,118	3,147
7	3,175	3,203	3,232	3,260	3,289	3,317	3,345	3,374	3,402	3,430	3,459	3,487	3,515	3,544	3,572	3,600
8	3,629	3,657	3,685	3,714	3,742	3,770	3,799	3,827	3,856	3,884	3,912	3,941	3,969	3,997	4,026	4,054
9	4,082	4,111	4,139	4,167	4,196	4,224	4,252	4,281	4,309	4,337	4,366	4,394	4,423	4,451	4,479	4,508
10	4,536	4,564	4,593	4,621	4,649	4,678	4,706	4,734	4,763	4,791	4,819	4,848	4,876	4,904	4,933	4,961
11	4,990	5,018	5,046	5,075	5103	5,131	5,160	5,188	5,216	5,245	5,273	5,301	5,330	5,358	5,386	5,415
12	5,443	5,471	5,500	5,528	5,557	5,585	5,613	5,642	5,670	5,698	5,727	5,755	5,783	5,812	5,840	5,868

Conversion of Centimeters to Inches					
Centimeters	Inches	Centimeters	Inches	Centimeters	Inches
25.4	10	43.2	17	61.0	24
26.7	10½	44.4	17½	62.2	24½
27.9	11	45.7	18	63.5	25
29.2	11½	47.0	18½	64.8	25½
30.5	12	48.3	19	66.1	26
31.8	12½	49.5	19½	67.4	26½
33.0	13	50.8	20	68.7	27
34.3	13½	52.1	20½	69.9	27½
35.6	14	53.3	21	71.2	28
36.8	14½	54.6	21½	72.5	28½
38.1	15	55.9	22	73.8	29
39.4	15½	57.2	22½	75.1	29½
40.6	16	58.4	23	76.4	30
41.9	16½	59.7	23½	77.6	30½

Conversion of Temperature (Fahrenheit and Celsius)	
Under most circumstances, a normal target range for a newborn's temperature is about 36.5°C to 37.5°C (97.7°F–99.5°F).	
Fahrenheit	Celsius
96.1	35.6
96.4	35.8
96.8	36.0
97.7	36.5
98.6	37.0
99.5	37.5
100.4	38.0
101.3	38.5
102.2	39.0
103.1	39.5
104.0	40.0
104.9	40.5
105.8	41.0
106.7	41.5
107.6	42.0

Apgar Scoring

Sign	0	1	2
Heart rate	Absent	<100	>100
Breathing	Absent	Weak	Strong cry
Color	Blue	Body pink; arms and legs blue	Pink
Tone	Limp	Some flexion	Well flexed
Reflexes	None	Grimace	Cough or sneeze

Derived from Apgar V. A proposal for a new method of evaluation of the newborn infant. *Curr Res Anesth Analg.* 1953;32(4):260–267. Reprinted with permission.

Expanded Apgar Score

Gestational Age _____ weeks

Sign	0	1	2	1 min	5 min	10 min	15 min	20 min
Color	Blue or pale	Acrocyanotic	Completely pink					
Heart rate	Absent	<100/min	>100/min					
Reflex irritability	No response	Grimace	Cry or active withdrawal					
Muscle tone	Limp	Some flexion	Active motion					
Respiration	Absent	Weak cry, hypoventilation	Good, crying					
			TOTAL					

Comments	Resuscitation					
		1	5	10	15	20
	Min					
	Oxygen					
	PPV/NCPAP					
	ETT					
	Chest compressions					
	Epinephrine					

Abbreviations: ETT, endotracheal tube; PPV/NCPAP, positive-pressure ventilation/nasal continuous positive airway pressure.
From American Academy of Pediatrics Committee on Fetus and Newborn, American College of Obstetricians and Gynecologists Committee on Obstetric Practice. The Apgar score. *Pediatrics.* 2006;117(4):1444–1447. Reprinted with permission from: The Apgar score. Committee Opinion No. 644. American College of Obstetricians and Gynecologists. *Obstet Gynecol.* 2015;126e:e52–e55.

Index